KT-130-016

Gower College Swansea

Gorseinon : Swansea : SA4 6RD Tel: (01792) 890731
This resource is **YOUR RESPONSIBILITY** and is due for
return/renewal on or before the last date shown.

CLASS NO. 616.89 BUR   ACC. NO. GCS027249

10 NOV 2017	2 6 FEB 2016
2 8 JUN 2018	
19 OCT 2023	

RETURN OR RENEW - DON'T PAY FINES

Very Short Introductions available now:

27249

GOWER COLLEGE SWANSEA
LEARNING RESOURCE CENTRE
GORSEINON
SWANSEA SA4 6RD

Tom Burns

PSYCHIATRY

A Very Short Introduction

ACC. No: GCS 027249
GOWER COLLEGE SWANSEA
LEARNING RESOURCE CENTRE

CLASS No: 616.89 BUR

OXFORD
UNIVERSITY PRESS

OXFORD

UNIVERSITY PRESS

Great Clarendon Street, Oxford OX2 6DP

Oxford University Press is a department of the University of Oxford.
It furthers the University's objective of excellence in research, scholarship,
and education by publishing worldwide in

Oxford New York

Auckland Cape Town Dar es Salaam Hong Kong Karachi
Kuala Lumpur Madrid Melbourne Mexico City Nairobi
New Delhi Shanghai Taipei Toronto

With offices in

Argentina Austria Brazil Chile Czech Republic France Greece
Guatemala Hungary Italy Japan Poland Portugal Singapore
South Korea Switzerland Thailand Turkey Ukraine Vietnam

Oxford is a registered trade mark of Oxford University Press
in the UK and in certain other countries

Published in the United States
by Oxford University Press Inc., New York

© Tom Burns 2006

The moral rights of the author have been asserted
Database right Oxford University Press (maker)

First published as a Very Short Introduction 2006

All rights reserved. No part of this publication may be reproduced,
stored in a retrieval system, or transmitted, in any form or by any means,
without the prior permission in writing of Oxford University Press,
or as expressly permitted by law, or under terms agreed with the appropriate
reprographics rights organizations. Enquiries concerning reproduction
outside the scope of the above should be sent to the Rights Department,
Oxford University Press, at the address above

You must not circulate this book in any other binding or cover
and you must impose this same condition on any acquirer

British Library Cataloguing in Publication Data

Data available

Library of Congress Cataloging in Publication Data

Data available

Typeset by RefineCatch Ltd, Bungay, Suffolk
Printed in Great Britain by
Ashford Colour Press Ltd., Gosport, Hants

ISBN 978-0-19-280727-4

Contents

27249

Preface

The current preference is for emphasizing that psychiatry is 'just another branch of medicine' like cardiology or oncology. In part this is to try and make psychiatry properly respectable by highlighting its scientific credentials, its commitment to precise diagnoses and evidence-based treatments, increasing its status within medicine and in society generally. It is also to reduce the stigma which has always been associated with mental illnesses. Stressing that these are illnesses like any other illness ('mental illnesses are brain diseases') should reduce prejudice experienced by sufferers and the sense of responsibility and shame felt by so many patients and families. We don't feel ashamed or blame ourselves if a family member develops arthritis, so why do we if they become depressed? It is against this backdrop of unnecessary additional suffering that the medical legitimacy of psychiatry is, quite rightly, stressed.

But it is not that simple. Psychiatry *is* different. Even those of us who work in it are treated as different. I am often asked, only half-joking, whether we become psychiatrists because we are odd or did we become odd as a result of being psychiatrists. The *New Yorker Magazine* produces compilations of its cartoons and there are invariably so many about psychiatrists that they regularly warrant their own volume.

Psychiatry can also inspire fear. It is, after all, the only branch of medicine which can force treatment on individuals. Special laws exist in all developed countries, both to protect the mentally ill against punishment but also to force them to have treatment. There appears to be a remarkable consensus about the reality and importance of mental illnesses despite, as will be clear throughout this book, the absence of simple objective definitions of them.

There is a fascination about psychiatry that goes beyond the natural curiosity about how the body or mind works. Psychoanalysts have suggested that this fascination (often mixed with fear) is because mental illnesses act out our own inner dramas. We see the depression we are struggling with and containing displayed before us, or individuals losing control when we may fear or secretly long to let go and shed our inhibitions.

There is certainly some truth in this. As I will explore in Chapter 1 the illnesses psychiatry deals with are diagnosed on the basis of experiences and feelings so familiar to us all. Yet they convey a sense of 'difference' at the same time. We find ourselves identifying with the descriptions, yet aware that some important threshold has been crossed. Psychiatry's increasing scientific sophistication has sharpened that threshold with enormous advances in consistency of diagnosis. However, Chapter 6 questions this increased certainty which brings some undesired consequences.

Psychiatry is, like all medicine, a pragmatic problem-solving activity. It draws on scientific theories but is not derived from them or constrained by them. Unlike psychology or physics, psychiatry cannot be explained 'top-down' from theories. Psychiatry has been formed by the illnesses that it has been required (and agreed) to treat and further shaped by the treatments it had available at the time. Consequently Chapter 1 includes descriptions of schizophrenia and manic depression and how these diseases and the care they received moulded the fledgling profession. The development of psychiatry is dependent on the values and structures of the societies that fostered it. It is almost impossible to understand current practices without understanding some of that history which is covered in Chapters 2 and 3. Similarly, the now relatively neglected contribution of psychoanalysis and psychotherapy is addressed in Chapter 4.

Chapters 5 and 6 deal with the controversies that have raged around and within psychiatry ever since it first emerged as a profession. It is a fair criticism of this book that it devotes more space to these than to the undeniable advances. I could have dwelt more on psychiatry's advances in new drugs, psychological treatments, and working practices which have made an enormous contribution to human welfare. Those who want to know more about these will easily find them elsewhere (increasingly on the web). I do not want to suggest any scepticism about the progress that psychiatry has made and is making. Psychiatry and the neurosciences are making remarkable strides.

I have devoted so much space to the controversial aspects of psychiatry for two reasons. First, because there are real philosophical and ethical differences between mental and physical illnesses that won't go away simply because we want them to. Nor will technological advances obliterate these tensions; rather, as explored in Chapter 6, more effective treatments may sharpen them. The challenge for psychiatry in the 21st century may be particularly acute in ethical and social questions posed by increasingly sophisticated and powerful treatments of the mind. Secondly, psychiatry is the arena where many of the big questions of the time – philosophical, political, and social – have to be hammered out in the crucible of real human relations and suffering. The philosophical debate about free will and determinism comes alive in the courtroom arguments about a psychiatric defence or in policy decisions about the management of psychopaths. The politics of power and social control drove the dismantling of the asylums and now frames the debate on compulsory treatment. The mind–brain dichotomy hovers throughout. The sustained battering from the anti-psychiatrists in the 1960s and 1970s (Chapter 5) raised the right (indeed, they would say the existential *obligation*) to be different.

So welcome to an area of medicine that is both mysterious and exciting as advances in brain sciences continually bump up against the messy reality of human beings. It is an activity which despite the scanners and designer drugs still rests on establishing trusting personal relationships. And lastly welcome to a pursuit that keeps challenging us about what it is to be truly human; continually reminding us of those unresolved philosophical issues (free will, mind–body dualism, personal autonomy versus social obligations) that we usually push to the back of our minds in order to get on with life.

List of illustrations

The publisher and the author apologize for any errors or omissions in the above list. If contacted they will be pleased to rectify these at the earliest opportunity.

Chapter 1
What is psychiatry?

The only normal people are the ones you don't know very well.

All of us know someone who has been troubled (anxious, depressed, or confused). Most of us have felt that way ourselves sometimes (adolescence is often a particular time of self-doubt and unhappiness). At these times our emotions may be overwhelming, unpredictable, and impossible to control and our thoughts strange and bizarre.

Does this mean that we have been mentally ill or need to see a psychiatrist? Luckily the answer for most of us is no. Yet when we read about psychiatry what we find described are experiences remarkably similar to these. Psychiatry is fascinating because it deals with consciousness, choice, motivation, free will, relationships – indeed everything that makes us human. While it is often cloaked in forbidding jargon ('affect' instead of mood, 'anxiety' instead of worry, 'phobia' rather than fear, 'cognition' instead of thinking) the conditions described are still instantly recognizable.

This is one of the persisting paradoxes about psychiatry that will recur throughout this book – that its subject is simultaneously firmly rooted in common human experience and yet is somehow 'that bit different'. We recognize similar experiences to our own in what the patient describes. They are immediately familiar to us, yet these familiar experiences are used to diagnose disorders quite outside our experience. Hopefully by the end of this book you will understand this dilemma better but I can't promise to resolve it for you. It's been argued about since psychiatry came into being and the argument still goes on. However, it may be best to start by defining what psychiatry is (and what it is not) before returning to the philosophical and political controversies that attend it.

All the 'psychs': psychology, psychotherapy, psychoanalysis, and psychiatry

'Psyche' is the Greek word for mind. All these four terms describe different approaches to understanding and helping individuals with psychological and emotional (mental) problems. There is lots of overlap, and sometimes the work done by the same highly qualified individual can be described by several of these terms, so it is not surprising that people confuse them. However, there are differences and getting them clear will help clarify what psychiatry is.

Psychology

Psychology is the study of human thought and behaviour. It originated just over a century ago from a tradition of introspective philosophy (trying to understand the minds of others by understanding our own) and is now a firmly established science. Psychology is studied at school and as an undergraduate course at university. It encompasses the study and understanding of mental processes in all their aspects and it has many branches. *Experimental psychologists* conduct experiments to explore the very basics of mental functioning (perception, memory, arousal, risk-taking, etc.). Indeed experimental psychologists do not restrict themselves exclusively to humans but study animals both in their own right and as models to understand human behaviour. Experimental psychology is generally considered a 'hard science' which follows the same scientific principles of investigation as physics or chemistry.

There are several professions stemming from psychology (e.g. *educational psychologists, industrial psychologists, forensic psychologists*). *Clinical psychologists* have postgraduate training in abnormal psychology and use this understanding to help people deal with their problems. The most obvious early example of this approach was the application of learning theory (i.e. consistent rewards and punishments to shape behaviour) in behaviour therapy. Behaviour therapy has been particularly successful in helping disturbed children or those with learning difficulties to modify their behaviour. It works without requiring a detailed understanding of the issues by the patient. Psychological treatments have, of course, become much more sophisticated and currently one of the most successful and widely practised psychotherapies (cognitive behaviour therapy) has been developed by clinical psychologists and is provided mainly by them. Clinical psychologists are essential members of all modern mental health ('psychiatric') services.

Psychoanalysis

Psychoanalysis is the method of treating neurotic disorders developed by Sigmund Freud towards the end of the 19th century in Vienna. In psychoanalysis the patient is encouraged to relax and say the first thing that comes into their mind ('free association') and to pay attention to their dreams and to the irrational aspects of their thinking. Freud was convinced that his patients suffered because they tried to keep unconscious (repress) thoughts and feelings that were unacceptable to them and that doing so caused their neurotic symptoms. The analyst listens carefully to what is said and over time begins to detect patterns and clues to these 'conflicts'. By sharing these insights he helps the patient confront and resolve them. Psychoanalysis is intensive and very long with patients traditionally coming for an hour a day up to five times a week for several years. Psychoanalysis is the origin of the cartoon image of the bearded psychiatrist sitting behind the patient lying on the couch.

Although Freud was a doctor there is no requirement for psychoanalysts to be medically trained. In America (where psychoanalysis has always had its most powerful presence) analysts were usually also psychiatrists but this is now increasingly the exception. Even when medically trained, analysts rarely use their medical knowledge – they make a virtue of not 'interfering' beyond the analysis. There are several schools of psychoanalysis developed by disciples of Freud (e.g. Jung, Adler, Klein) and some have become quite remote from the original model (e.g. Reich, Lacan). Psychoanalysis has had enormous influence beyond psychiatry, particularly in literature and the arts. Terms like 'Freudian' and 'Freudian slip' are part of everyday speech. However, because psychoanalysis lacks firm scientific evidence of its efficacy, it is increasingly marginalized in modern psychiatric practice.

Psychotherapy

It soon became clear that there was more to psychoanalysis than Freud's original remote and neutral exploration of the unconscious. The relationships formed in this intense treatment were themselves found to be influential. Analysts began to explore these relationships and experimented with more active approaches and with different types of therapy (time-limited therapies, more structured therapies, therapies in groups and in families, etc.). These psychological approaches, in which the relationship was used actively through talking to promote self-awareness and change, are broadly understood as 'psychotherapy'. Most of the early psychotherapies leant heavily on Freud's theories (often called 'psychodynamic psychotherapy' to emphasize the impact of thoughts and feelings over time) but several of the newer ones do not. These (e.g. non-directive counselling, existential psychotherapy, transactional analysis, cognitive analytical and cognitive behaviour therapy) draw on a range of theoretical backgrounds.

What they all have in common is that they use communication

within a formalized and secure relationship to explore difficulties and find ways of either adapting to them or overcoming them. Most psychodynamic psychotherapies also require (like psychoanalysis) that the therapist undergoes a treatment themselves as part of the training. Psychoanalysis remains very tightly controlled, by defining strictly who becomes a psychoanalyst, but psychotherapy is a loose concept. Some schools of psychotherapy are strict about whom they admit but the title 'psychotherapist' could, until recently, be used by anyone. Most psychotherapists are not psychiatrists although most psychiatrists have some psychotherapy training and skills. Some psychiatrists even work mainly as psychotherapists. Chapter 4 is devoted to psychoanalysis and psychotherapy.

What is psychiatry?

So if it is not psychology and not psychoanalysis or psychotherapy, what is psychiatry? There are overlaps with the other 'psychs' but there are some fundamental differences. First and foremost psychiatry is a branch of *medicine* – you can't become a psychiatrist without first qualifying as a doctor. Having qualified, the future psychiatrist spends several years in further training. He or she works with, and learns about, mental illnesses in exactly the same way that a dermatologist would train by treating patients with skin disorders or an obstetrician by delivering babies. Within medicine, psychiatry is simply defined as that branch which deals with 'mental illnesses' (nowadays often called 'psychiatric disorders').

Medicine is fundamentally a pragmatic endeavour. While drawing heavily on the basic biological sciences and scientific methods, the ultimate test of whether a treatment is right is if the patient gets better. We don't *have* to know how the treatment works. Therefore the definition of psychiatry is not based on theory, as in psychology or psychoanalysis, but on practice. Whatever is viewed as mental illnesses (and this has changed over time), and whatever treatments are available for these illnesses, will determine what a psychiatrist is, and what he or she does.

What is a mental illness?

There is a marked circularity about this ('a psychiatrist is someone who diagnoses and treats psychiatric disorders', 'psychiatric disorders are those conditions which are diagnosed and treated by psychiatrists'). There has been endless controversy about the reliability of psychiatric diagnoses and even whether or not mental illnesses exist at all (Chapter 5). It is worth spending a little time on why psychiatric diagnoses are so controversial both because it keeps cropping up and also because the same issues are fundamental to all medicine although rarely as striking.

The subjectivity of diagnosis

The hallmark of the psychiatrist's trade is the interview. We make our diagnoses (and still conduct much of our treatment) in face-to-face discussions with patients. We take a careful history (as do all doctors) but then, instead of, or sometimes in addition to, conducting a physical examination (feeling the abdomen, taking the pulse, listening through a stethoscope) we conduct what is called a 'mental state exam'. In this we probe deeper into what is worrying the patient, their mood, way of thinking, etc. Some of this involves simply noting what the patient reports (that they are hearing strange sounds or that they panic every time they think of going out) but some involves us in constructing an understanding of what they are going through using 'directed empathy'. Directed empathy means actively putting ourselves in their shoes, understanding what they are feeling and thinking, even if they have difficulty in expressing it. For instance we may come to the conclusion that a patient who recounts a series of vindictive acts carried out against them by strangers and friends alike is, in fact, excessively suspicious (paranoid) leading to misinterpretation of common events.

This ability to piece together how other people experience things and what they are feeling is an essential human capacity.

6

Understanding how others see the world from their perspective (often called having 'a theory of mind') is so important that its absence, as in Autism or Asperger's Syndrome, is a profound handicap. Psychiatrists train up this skill and, because of increasing familiarity with the range of disorders, can use it actively to understand the confused and confusing experiences that patients recount to them.

Diagnoses based on a patient's mental state contain no concrete evidence for the diagnosis – there are no blood tests or x-ray pictures. A written list of what is said or a detailed description of the behaviour (e.g. the diagnostic criteria for depression) are only part of the process. Psychiatric diagnoses rely on making a judgement about *why* someone is doing something, not just the observation of *what* they are doing. Hence the criticism that they are not scientific; they are not 'objective'. Take the example of an elderly man who is profoundly depressed. He may not say that he is depressed but instead complain of tiredness, aches and pains, poor sleep and feelings of guilt. As he deteriorates he may lie unmoving all day or even not speak at all. A psychiatrist will probably interpret his immobility as a feature of depression. In doing this (usually supported by the other clues) he hypothesizes that the immobility is a result of despair and hopelessness. There are lots of other possible causes of immobility (or 'stupor' in its most extreme form) and the psychiatrist distinguishes depressive stupor from those caused by hormonal or neurological problems by building up a picture of the patient's mental state, i.e. *why* he is not moving or communicating.

Imposing categories on dimensions

The range of human variation is something we cherish. We would hate a world where everyone had the same personality, where there were no sensitive individuals, no moody individuals, no brave brash ones, etc. Similarly life without emotional variation would be intolerable. Aldous Huxley's book *Brave New World* (where everyone was able to remain constantly content by taking a drug called 'Soma') was a nightmare scenario, not a utopia. Normal

Diagnostic Criteria for Major Depressive Episode (DSM IV*)

Five (or more) of the following present during the same 2 week period and is a change from previous functioning; at least one of the symptoms is either (1) depressed mood or (2) loss of interest or pleasure.

Depressed mood most of the day, nearly every day (e.g. feels sad or empty) or observed by others (e.g. appears tearful).

Markedly diminished interest or pleasure in all, or almost all, activities most of the day, nearly every day (subjective account or observation).

Significant weight loss or weight gain (more than 5% of body weight in a month), or decrease or increase in appetite nearly every day.

Insomnia or hypersomnia nearly every day.

Agitation or retardation nearly every day (observable by others).

Fatigue or loss of energy nearly every day.

Feelings of worthlessness or excessive or inappropriate guilt nearly every day.

Diminished ability to think or concentrate, or indecisiveness, nearly every day.

Recurrent thoughts of death, recurrent suicidal ideation.

The symptoms do not meet criteria for a Mixed Episode.

The symptoms cause clinically significant distress or impairment in social or occupational functioning.

The symptoms not due to drug abuse, medication, or a general medical condition.

The symptoms are not better accounted for by bereavement.

*DSM IV = the fourth version of the Diagnostic and Statistical Manual produced by the American Psychiatric Association. A codification of diagnostic criteria for psychiatric disorders used worldwide. 'Statistical' refers to the use of these categories to record diagnoses and treatment.

intensities of sadness (e.g. in grief) or fear (e.g. in a house fire) match anything to be found in mental illnesses. There is no consistent cut-off, no absolute distinction between the normal and the abnormal – it is not a simple matter of degree. Even hearing voices when there is nobody about (auditory hallucinations) occurs in 'normal' people. Research in the Netherlands found a significant number of healthy people who regularly 'hear voices'; widows and widowers regularly hear the voice of their dead partner quite clearly (and usually find it comforting). So how can the psychiatrist claim that hallucinations are symptoms of mental illness?

Medical practice involves pattern recognition. For most disorders there is a set of symptoms and signs that characterize it. Not all have to be present to make the diagnosis, although obviously that makes it easier. If some of the symptoms are very prominent then we hardly need to confirm the others, but if none is very striking we will seek to complete the picture. The intensity and duration of the symptoms also matter (how long the anxiety lasts, how persistent and disruptive the voices). Judgements must accommodate cultural differences. Northern Europeans are usually much less emotionally demonstrative than Southern Europeans so the thresholds for concern about expressions of distress may vary, for example, between a Finn and an Italian.

Traditionally medical training involved seeing as many patients as possible to learn these patterns within the normal range of expression. More recently diagnostic systems have become more formalized, often requiring some features absolutely and then a selection of others as shown in the current diagnostic criteria for depression. This has certainly improved consistency but the process is still the same. In this example 'lowered mood' is treated as a yes/no, present/absent quality, when we all know that mood varies continuously between people and over time. Psychiatric diagnoses require the imposition of *categories* (yes/no, present/absent) onto what are really *dimensions* (a little/quite a bit/a bit more/quite a lot/too much).

This is very obvious in psychiatry but it is certainly not unique to it. Our popular view of illnesses is usually based on the examples of infectious diseases or surgical trauma – you've either got an infection or you have not, your leg is either broken or it is not. There is no ambiguity and no need for agreement or consensus. However, few illnesses are that straightforward. Even the infection example is not that simple – you can find the same bacteria that cause pneumonia in lots of perfectly healthy people. The diagnosis is not made just by finding the bacteria but by finding them in the presence of a fever and cough. Even objective, verifiable data don't always resolve the issue. What is considered 'pathological' will change depending on changing knowledge about diseases and available treatments. Just as improved treatments have led us to lower the threshold for depression so the diagnosis of disorders as apparently concrete and measurable as diabetes and high blood pressure is constantly redefined.

So psychiatry is not for the faint-hearted or those who need too much intellectual security. It is, of all the branches of medicine, the one that most clearly exposes the processes behind making a diagnosis. The language is revealing – doctors 'make' diagnoses, they impose their patterns rather than simply discovering them. It is also the branch of medicine which most explicitly acknowledges the impact of social considerations on its practice. Both the definitions of disorders used by psychiatrists and their expression in individuals are moulded by the social context. For example, modern society identifies and treats battle stress or shell-shock in war as a psychiatric disorder whereas a century ago we punished it as cowardice. Young adults at the start of the 21st century will seek help for their problems in a manner utterly unrecognizable to how their stoical grandparents would have done. This doesn't make psychiatry particularly unscientific or unreliable (psychiatric diagnoses are about as reliable as those in medicine overall). However, it reminds us that, like medicine, it remains (despite current wishful thinking) both an art and a science and draws from both social and physical sciences.

The scope of psychiatry – psychoses, neuroses, and personality problems

Psychiatrists deal with a wide range of problems. The most severe disorders are often referred to as 'functional' (or non-organic) psychoses and include schizophrenia and manic depression (now usually referred to as bipolar disorder). The distinction into organic and non-organic is rather messy but still useful. Although we are increasingly convinced that there are organic (usually brain) changes underlying most of these illnesses, 'organic' is reserved for those psychoses arising from another, usually very obvious, disease. These include a range of causes of confusion and mental disturbance such as injury, chronic intoxication, and dementia plus a range of more short-lived physical causes such as severe infections, hormone imbalances, etc. Functional psychoses are the conditions to which the older term 'madness' was applied. People with these were said to have 'lost their reason'. Overall they affect nearly 3 per cent of the population at some stage in their life. So while they are not very common they are not that rare – about one person in an average secondary school class will suffer a psychotic illness in the course of their adult life.

The defining characteristic of psychosis is the loss of insight into the personal origins of the strange experiences. The patient loses the ability to 'reality test' – to check his or her terrifying or melancholic thoughts and feelings against external reality and judge them. He can't think 'I'm blaming myself for everything and can't see a way forward because I'm depressed.' Rather, he thinks 'I feel this way as punishment for what I've done and there is no future.' He may actively deny that he is ill and resist the attempts of those around him to balance these misinterpretations. Being so fixated on internal experiences, unable to modify them despite evidence to the contrary, is often referred to as 'losing contact with reality'. He denies that he is ill and cannot see that family or mental health staff want to help. Psychoses can be terrifying experiences with high levels of anxiety and distress. The two major psychoses have so defined the development of psychiatry that it is worth our time now to learn about them in some detail.

Schizophrenia

Schizophrenia is probably the most severe of all the mental illnesses. It does not mean split personality – Dr Jekyll and Mr Hyde was not a case of schizophrenia. The name was introduced by a Swiss doctor, Eugen Bleuler, in 1911 to emphasize the disintegration ('splitting') of mental functioning. It affects just under 1 per cent of the population worldwide and usually starts in early adulthood (during the 20s) although it can occur as early as adolescence. While it affects men and women in equal numbers, men often become ill earlier and fare worse. The prominent features are hallucinations, delusions, thought disorder, social withdrawal, and self-neglect.

Hallucinations are 'sensory experiences without stimuli'. Far and away the most common are auditory hallucinations – hearing voices which talk to the patient or talk about them. Seeing things is not uncommon (though rarely as complete or persistent as auditory hallucinations) and many patients have strange physical sensations of things happening in their body. Hallucinations are not simply imagining our thoughts as a voice in the head – most of us do that. They are experienced with the full force of an external event, fully awake in broad daylight; there is no 'as if' quality to them and the patient believes they are entirely real.

Delusions are 'firm, fixed false ideas that are inconsistent with the patient's culture'. Deciding that something is a delusion requires more understanding of context than identifying a hallucination. The striking thing about delusions is the *intensity* with which they are held and how impervious they are to rational argument or proof to the contrary. The patient has no doubt either about their truth or about their importance.

The world is now a very culturally mixed place and a judgement often has to be made about whether ideas are really that odd for any particular individual. For example, two quite different patients described to me their conviction that there were invisible force-fields traversing their living rooms which affected them. The first was a young 'New Age' woman preoccupied with Ley lines, Druidic culture, and mysticism. No illness here. The second was a retired schoolmistress who was convinced the force fields were electric, originated from her neighbour and represented an attempt to influence her sexually. This latter is a classic delusion in late-onset schizophrenia and had resulted in her exposing the electrical wiring in her house to get at the source. In schizophrenia delusions are commonly persecutory ('paranoid') and the source of the persecution (e.g. police, communists, the devil, freemasons) varies across time and place.

Thought disorder as a symptom is often considered particularly characteristic of schizophrenia. Schizophrenia differs from other psychiatric disorders in that not only is the *content* of thought often unusual (not surprising given the impact of hallucinations and delusions) but its logical and grammatical *form* can be disturbed. With thought disorder it can sometimes be simply impossible to understand what the patient means, although each individual word can be understood. At its most extreme, conversation can be totally incomprehensible with lots of invented words and jumbled sentences. More often, however, sentences appear logical but lead nowhere or can't be recalled. Where they can be recalled, despite repeating and exploring them, they simply can't be understood.

Obviously you have to be careful before diagnosing thought disorder that it isn't just a case of the patient being cleverer than you or knowing more (both always a possibility). However, recovered patients often tell us that at these times they did not feel fully in control of their thoughts. They may have experienced thoughts being directly inserted into, or withdrawn from, their minds or that they became suddenly aware of new connections between things that were uniquely revealed to them. This sense of *unique new meanings* is rare in other disorders and can lead to words being used in different and puzzling ways. A patient who had just 'become aware' that the colour green 'meant intimacy' (didn't imply intimacy or wasn't associated with intimacy but 'meant' intimacy) constructed sentences using it this way fully convinced that we also understood it.

Withdrawal and self-neglect are probably among the most distressing and disabling features of schizophrenia. Bleuler, who first used the term, thought that withdrawal from engagement with others was central to the disorder and he used the term 'autism' to describe it. Although Bleuler was the first to use the term schizophrenia he was not the one who identified the condition. Kraepelin did that in 1896, but he called it 'Dementia Praecox' based on the gradual deterioration over time which he thought always occurred. Both these early researchers considered what we now call the 'positive symptoms' (hallucinations, delusions, and thought disorder) to be secondary to the core process of withdrawal and turning inward – the so-called 'negative symptoms'.

During the last half-century, with the development of antipsychotic drugs (which target these positive symptoms), we have tended to see it the other way round – assuming that the negative symptoms are a consequence of the positive ones. After each acute episode recovered patients did not get fully better, they were that bit less engaged, less interested in themselves or the world around them. However, the pendulum is swinging back with more attention to these negative symptoms, not least because our drug treatments are much less effective with them.

Kraepelin was very gloomy about schizophrenia and believed that virtually no patients really got better, but Bleuler was more positive and the truth lies closer to him. It is a fluctuating illness and most patients have several bouts. About a quarter probably recover well, having only one or two episodes. Most, however, have several episodes and take longer to get better after each one and rarely get back 100 per cent to where they started. A small proportion of patients have a very poor outcome and spend much of their adult lives overwhelmingly handicapped by the disease, unable to live independently. Modern treatments, particularly antipsychotic drugs, mean that most patients only come into hospital for a few weeks or months when they relapse, not the years that characterized pre-war mental hospitals. Schizophrenia runs in families and there is little real argument any longer that genetics play a role (see Chapter 5).

Manic depressive disorder (bipolar disorder)

Modern psychiatry owes its intellectual framework to Kraepelin's distinction between schizophrenia and manic depressive illness. This is now renamed bipolar disorder, the term used from here on. During Kraepelin's time mental hospitals took whoever was sent to them; some got better but most didn't. There was not that much attention to diagnosis other than perhaps distinguishing the learning disabled from the psychotic. Kraepelin noted that one group of patients alternated through several periods of profound disturbances – sometimes agitated and sometimes withdrawn and depressed. What distinguished them most from the schizophrenia patients (which he called 'dementia praecox') was that they made full recoveries between episodes and more of them eventually left hospital. It was the *course* of the illness rather than its symptoms that impressed him (see Chapter 2).

Bipolar patients *can* have all the same symptoms as in schizophrenia (hallucinations, delusions, thought disorder, etc.) although these occur only in the most severe forms of mania and depression. However these symptoms are accompanied by a profound disturbance of mood – either depression or elation. It is this elation that is called mania (or often hypomania). The change in mood overshadows all else in this condition. In the depressed phase the patient suffers from severe depression and may be suicidal. In the elated phase the patient is overactive and bursting with confidence and energy. Hypomanic patients can be very destructive to themselves – spending money they haven't got and behaving in an uninhibited manner (drinking too much, being sexually overactive without thought for the consequences, driving too fast, etc.). The psychotic symptoms, where they occur, reflect the mood. If the patient is depressed hallucinations will be critical and persecuting, if elated the hallucinations praise and encourage. Depressive delusions are usually of guilt and worthlessness and hypomanic delusions are expansive and grandiose: 'I'm going to be asked to advise the president about foreign policy', 'My paintings are worth millions'.

In less extreme forms of hypomania patients can be very entertaining, often talking fast ('pressure of speech'), punning and making humorous associations between ideas ('flight of ideas'). Many famous entertainers and artists have suffered from bipolar disorder and acknowledge that they get their inspiration when they are 'high'. It can be difficult to be certain about diagnosis in some of the milder forms of hypomania because it usually lacks the 'strangeness' of the schizophrenic episode. The main disturbance is one of judgement – we would all like to spend more money or hope that our paintings are worth more than they are. Often the diagnosis needs friends and family members to be able to confirm that this is not how the person usually is. A rather flamboyant, flirty TV executive was brought to the clinic by her worried mother. The story was not, in itself, that remarkable – some rather torrid love affairs with work colleagues, recreational drug use in night clubs, and some incidences of rudeness to her boss and absences from work. There are lots of media people who conduct their lives like this. What was decisive was her mother's description of how normally she was an over-conscientious, rather anxious woman and that this was completely out of character. The mother was alert to the issue because her late husband had also suffered such episodes.

Like schizophrenia, bipolar disorder also affects just under 1 per cent of the population, it runs in families, it starts in early adult life (though usually later than schizophrenia) and males and females are affected about equally. Although the elated phases are more dramatic depression is more frequent and persistent. The depressive phase of bipolar disorder is not easily distinguishable from the much more common disorder of clinical depression.

Treatment of psychotic disorders

This is not a book to deal in any detail with individual treatments. Treatments in psychiatry, like any other branch of medicine, are evolving so fast that any description here would soon be out of date.

A range of drugs have been developed since the 1950s ('antipsychotics' such as chlorpromazine, haloperidol, risperidone, clozapine, olanzapine) which are effective in settling patients during the acute phases of schizophrenia. Unlike earlier drugs like barbiturates these are tranquillizing rather than sedative. They calm the mind without making the patient fall asleep (they do often have drowsiness as a side effect but that is not their purpose). Antipsychotics have revolutionized the treatment of acute psychotic episodes with calmer, shorter spells in hospital. Continuing on antipsychotics after recovery reduces the risk of further breakdowns, and most psychiatrists encourage schizophrenia patients to stay on them for many, many years ('maintenance treatment'). Obviously this is not easy as all drugs have some side effects and nobody likes taking them endlessly. With support, however, many patients do succeed in staying on them and suffer far fewer breakdowns.

Severe depressive episodes in bipolar patients can be treated either with antidepressants or, in extreme cases, with electro convulsive treatment (ECT). These are discussed below. There are also now a number of 'mood stabilizers' which are used in the maintenance treatment of bipolar disorder and significantly reduce the risk of breakdown. Drugs are certainly not the only treatments available for psychotic disorders (Chapter 3) but they are currently the cornerstone.

Compulsory treatment

Lack of insight can pose real risks of a psychotic patient harming himself or others as he tries to flee or defend himself from perceived threats or persecution. Because of this impairment in judgement about the need for treatment, and the very real risks during psychotic states, psychiatry has been the one branch of medicine where the patient's right to refuse treatment can be overruled. This is dealt with in more detail in Chapters 2 and 6. Provision for compulsory treatment is universal in psychiatric services and the overall principle seems generally accepted. The conditions under which it can be applied however (who imposes it, whether it is restricted to hospital care, whether there needs to be immediate risk of physical danger, etc.) vary enormously from country to country and reflect local values.

Compulsory detention for the severely mentally ill ('the furiously mad', Chapter 2) evolved before there were any effective treatments. It reflects a recognition that mental illness is not simply deviance ('mad' not 'bad'). Had it not been the case those at risk solely to themselves would have been left to their own devices and those presenting a risk to others would have been simply subject to the law. It was recognized in mental illnesses that the individual was changed from his normal self, and could change back. Detaining the patient served to protect him or her while the illness ran its course until they recovered ('were restored to reason'). Of course not everyone did get better but enough did to sustain the hope and justify the humanitarian protective impulse behind detention.

Depression and neurotic disorders

Not all psychiatric disorders involve the same break with reality found in psychoses. In fact the majority of patients seen by psychiatrists do not suffer from psychoses but from less devastating disorders. Most of these are characterized by persisting high levels of depression and anxiety. They used to be lumped together under the title of 'neuroses' but the term has become unfashionable in psychiatry. However, it is a useful term, albeit rather vague, and one that most people understand so it will be used here. Neuroses cause distress and suffering to those who have them and may not be at all obvious to others. They vary greatly in severity and many patients are able to lead normal lives (marrying and working) while coping with them. Some, however, can be as disabling as the psychoses.

Depression

Depression is the commonest psychiatric disorder and affects about 15 per cent of us in our lifetime. The World Health Organization ranks it second to heart disease as a cause of lifelong disability worldwide. It appears to be becoming more common (particularly in the developed world), although some of this may be better detection, greater public awareness, and greater willingness to seek help. Luckily, with the advent of antidepressants and the development of more effective psychological treatments (e.g. cognitive behaviour therapy), it usually gets better fairly quickly. Most patients are treated by their family doctor and only the most severe get referred to psychiatrists. A proportion of depressed patients eventually become diagnosed as having bipolar disorder but here we focus on the 'non-psychotic' group.

Depression is usually experienced as a profound sense of misery, a loss of hope in the future, and often associated with self-doubt and self-criticism. Tension and anxiety are very common, sleep is disturbed, and patients lose weight and find themselves unable to concentrate properly or get on with things. Tearfulness and thoughts of suicide are common and aches, pains, and health worries frequent. In more severe cases patients report 'feeling nothing' (being cold and empty, unable to enjoy anything) rather than sadness. Patients may also take to alcohol or drugs as self-medication, which almost always makes things worse. Depression differs from our normal periods of sadness by going on and on without relief, and the weight loss and poor sleep perpetuate it.

Depression is three times more common in women than men. Some people are constitutionally or temperamentally more at risk of developing it but it is clearly influenced by life circumstances. It is much more common in those living in poverty, those who are unemployed, live alone, have few friends or who have painful or disabling physical illnesses. Early loss of a mother and a difficult childhood are associated with an increased risk of becoming depressed as an adult. Depression is also more likely to follow from severe personal problems (relationship break ups, exam failure, job loss, etc.).

Helping people with depression almost always needs more than antidepressants (though these are very effective). Counselling, help to see a way forward, specific psychotherapy, and attention to ensuring a supportive social network are all needed. Understanding depression better has led to the recognition of just how important social networks and friendships are to people. These are not optional extras and few of us can survive without them. Providing such networks for young isolated mothers and their children in programmes such as Head Start in the US and Sure Start in the UK are national programmes that include strategies to prevent depression.

Most of us will experience some periods of depression in our lives with all of the features above. Most of us will get over them spontaneously and fairly quickly. Indeed, it is possible to think of depression as a necessary and useful human process – a period when we can work through loss, acknowledge it properly, and find a new balance. At such times it is appropriate to withdraw a bit into ourselves and some psychoanalysts consider the ability to be depressed as an essential step towards personal maturity. Certainly people who don't seem ever to be depressed strike us as different or odd. Psychiatrists have spent years trying to make a clear distinction between 'clinical depression' and 'normal depression' and, frankly, have failed. The difference is more one of degree than genetics or symptom pattern. If it goes on and on, or if the symptoms become unbearable, it needs to be treated; if it gets better on its own after a few weeks, then great.

Anxiety

Anxiety is fear spread thin. We've all experienced it and undoubtedly it is useful – a degree of anxiety is essential to keep us alert and get us to perform well – e.g. fear of failure gets us to work hard for exams. However psychological studies show that, while performance rises with anxiety up to a point, above a certain level our performance plummets. Anxiety disorders are probably about as common as depression but fewer people seek help for them. People with 'Generalized Anxiety Disorder' (GAD) are persistently over-anxious. Most of us experience similar anxiety levels from time to time, but in anxiety disorders it doesn't settle. GAD is exhausting and sufferers can't sleep, lose weight, and often can't concentrate. If it goes on a long time they may become depressed.

Phobic disorders are more dramatic and noticeable. A phobia means an exaggerated fear. Most of us have a phobia – so-called simple phobias start in childhood and are constant through life. Animal phobias are typical examples (spiders, mice, snakes). Mine is a height phobia – I can't climb towers or go near cliff edges. Most people live with their simple phobias unless they begin to interfere seriously with life (e.g. a flying phobia in someone whose job begins to require frequent travel, a needle phobia in a woman who becomes pregnant and needs to have blood tests). Simple phobias are remarkably easy to cure by behaviour therapy using 'graded exposure'. You get used to the feared object by following a preset scheme increasing the exposure while monitoring your own anxiety (e.g. start with holding a picture of a spider then hold a small dead one, a larger dead one, a living one in a glass, a living one free, and then a tarantula!).

Most of the phobias seen by psychiatrists are not simple phobias. They are either agoraphobia or social phobia. These start in adult life, are not constant (they are worse in times of stress), and can be quite disabling. Agoraphobia is not fear of open spaces as many think, but of crowds and crowded places. It comes from the Greek word *Agoros* for market place, not the Latin word *Ager* for field. Agoraphobia affects women much more and is associated with panic attacks and often leads to staying in and avoiding crowds. It is this 'avoidance' that makes the disorder continue. Panic attacks are awful (racing heart, sweating, a dry mouth, and conviction that one is going to faint, wet oneself, or even die). It is no surprise that people exit the situation as fast as possible and avoid it. The pity is that if they stayed they would soon realize that panic is very short-lived (a matter of minutes, not hours) and fades on its own. However when we rush off and the panic stops we become convinced that it was the getting away that stopped it and we don't learn that we can ride out the panic. The memory of the last panic starts to get us anxious as we approach the situation again and this 'fear of the fear' increases the likelihood of another attack.

Treatment is usually based on behaviour therapy, teaching the person how to stay with a panic attack and thereby reduce it. It is usually a bit more complicated than with simple phobias. Social phobia is an exaggerated anxiety on meeting people. There is some real controversy about whether this is a legitimate diagnosis or simply severe shyness, and particularly whether it should be treated with drugs (Chapter 6). In social phobia the problem is usually one of avoidance rather than panic and the treatment involves counselling to help develop techniques for dealing with social situations.

Obsessive compulsive disorder

Most of us have experienced obsessional behaviour as children – avoiding the cracks in the pavement to avoid catastrophic consequences is the commonest. Sportsmen and actors are notorious for such rituals – the tennis player who *has* to bounce the ball three times before serving, the leading lady who cannot play without something green in her costume. These superstitious behaviours have much in common with obsessive compulsive disorder (OCD). In this disorder the patient has to repeat activities or thoughts (classically hand washing or checking and counting rituals) a set number of times or in a set order to ward off anxiety or feared consequences. In the obsessional form (where there are often no external rituals) the problem is repetitive thoughts, often about awful outcomes (contamination with dirt or germs, or a fear of shouting out something blasphemous or offensive). The hallmark of OCD is that the thoughts or actions are *repeated, resisted,* and *distressing*. It isn't a harmless superstition or quirk but can dominate and ruin lives. Compulsive cleaners, for instance, end up exhausted because they are never finished cleaning over and over again. Obsessional ruminators can't hold down a job because they are distracted with repeating their thoughts or counting and may wear out their partners as they seek constant reassurance about their worries.

OCD tends to be associated with specific personality traits – neat, tidy, conscientious. Most of us recognize obsessional features in ourselves and yet the full disorder seems so bizarre. Indeed, sufferers are often slow to seek help because they consider it so strange and incomprehensible – they are embarrassed by it. It has been subject to psychological over-interpretation (Chapter 4) and only recently have effective treatments been developed (behaviour therapy and antidepressants in milder cases).

Hysterical disorders

Hysteria is no longer a fashionable term. In general use it often just means over-emotional (and usually in women) – 'Oh don't be so hysterical!' Hysterical disorders were originally thought to be restricted to women. *Hysteros* is the Greek word for womb and there were once fanciful theories of the symptoms being caused by the womb wandering within the body. In psychiatry it has played an important role – particularly in psychoanalysis (Chapter 4) which still gives the best explanation of it.

Hysterical disorders are most often striking physical or neurological symptoms for which no organic cause can be found. In 'conversion' disorders anxiety or conflict is expressed as ('converted into') a pain or disability. The most dramatic are paralyses or blindness. The patient insists that they cannot see or move their arm and yet all tests indicate that they 'really' can. In dissociative disorders patients deal with their conflicts by insisting that they are not in touch with some aspect of their mental functioning ('dissociating' from it). In the most extreme case an individual may insist they have multiple personalities and are not responsible for what different 'personalities' do. One of the surprising features of hysterical disorders is that the patient appears relatively content with what appear to others to be very frightening physical conditions. Charcot, the great 19th-century French neurologist, called this contentment 'la belle indifférence'.

Conversion and dissociation mechanisms are very common (and temporarily often very helpful) in times of enormous stress. Soldiers in war often carry on apparently calm under fire but afterwards have absolutely no memory of it. Most of us have developed a terrible headache or felt unwell inexplicably only later to realize that it was a way of avoiding something we couldn't face. In some cases we may doubt if the mechanism is really unconscious, as when it is used in a legal defence (e.g. automatism in murder trials).

Hysteria in adults is getting less common in more 'psychologically sophisticated' societies. In the First World War soldiers, who could not easily acknowledge their terror, developed shell shock (a coarse shaking of the hands and 'jumpiness') which was undoubtedly hysterical. They were genuinely unaware that (were 'unconscious of' the fact that) the fear of battle caused their symptoms. By the Second World War it was fully understood that soldiers could be terrified of battle. Those who could not cope did not develop shell shock but 'battle stress'. They felt the terror and could not function but recognized what it was and asked for help. They did not have to deny the fear and convert it into 'acceptable' symptoms such as tremor or paralysis. While conversion symptoms are relatively rare now in psychiatric wards they continue to be a significant issue in other medical specialties where the more neutral term 'somatization' is used. Treatment is usually based on identifying the stresses and helping the patient find other ways of dealing with them. Treatment of acute hysterical disorders with abreactions (i.e. giving a sedative drug and getting the patient to talk through the situation under its influence) was often amazingly dramatic and effective.

Personality disorders

We all have a personality. Personality is that collection of relatively permanent characteristics that makes us different from each other. It's generally how we first think of individuals or describe them. Psychiatrists inevitably became interested in personality. First because they have to distinguish between illness and personality (is this person suffering from a depression or are they always morose and pessimistic?). But they soon noted that there were personality types that were more commonly associated with some of the disorders they treated and for this reason they used the same or similar terms. The schizoid personality is rather distant and strange and the paranoid personality is over-sensitive and prone to suspicion. The hysterical is prone to intense fluctuating emotions, needing passionate relationships and to be the centre of attention, whereas the obsessional is careful and inflexible. The psychopathic personality (variously called sociopathic and antisocial) is not just a delinquent but is characterized by an absence of feeling for those around him or any sense of remorse. Their difference from ordinary criminals is such that prisons have as much difficulty dealing with them as do psychiatric hospitals.

The role of psychiatry in the treatment of extremes of personality, 'personality disorders' (PD) is controversial (Chapter 6) and most psychiatrists are sceptical that they have any specific cures. However, personality affects everything about us and so the treatment of any psychiatric disorder will require proper attention to personality. Different societies present problems for different personalities and the classification of personality disorders is changing. The difference between the sexes in the distribution of the two most prominent diagnoses is striking. Currently women are much more likely to be diagnosed with 'borderline' PD (fluctuating, intense emotions and difficult relationships, self-harm and low self-esteem, quite similar to the old-term 'hysterical' PD) and men with 'antisocial' PD (violence, delinquency, and impulsiveness quite similar to 'psychopathic' PD). It is not hard to see how these two disorders could be manifestations of the same personal alienation and disappointment but expressed as 'different' disorders because of how our culture moulds the behaviours of men and women.

Addictions

It is far from clear what psychiatry's role should be in the treatment of alcohol and drug abuse. Most people who abuse them do not have mental illnesses. However there are a number of compelling reasons why psychiatry is involved. People with mental health problems have a very much increased risk of turning to drink or drugs, possibly to dull the pain in their lives (particularly in depression and personality disorders). Drug and alcohol abuse also makes getting better much more difficult. It is almost impossible to recover fully from depression while drinking to excess and young schizophrenia patients who abuse drugs find it difficult to attain control of their illnesses.

Addictions can also *cause* mental illnesses. Severe alcohol abuse can lead to paranoid psychoses, delirium tremens, depression, and eventually dementia. Amphetamine and cocaine are associated with quite severe paranoid disorders which can result in violence; acute psychotic reactions are common with LSD and Ecstasy. In addition the poverty and social chaos associated with illegal drug use can lead to depression and despair. So psychiatry is inevitably involved with treating alcohol and drug misuse. However, whether psychiatry should lead it, or simply be one of a range of inputs available to help, can be debated, as can the benefit of classifying addictions as illnesses.

Suicide

Suicide is a tragic, but not infrequent, occurrence in psychiatry. About a quarter of those who commit suicide are in current contact with psychiatrists and in the UK two-thirds have consulted their GP in the last month (40 per cent in the last week). The psychiatric disorders with the highest risk for suicide are alcoholism and depression, although it is increasingly recognized as a long-term risk in psychotic disorders and anorexia nervosa. Although suicide attempts are more common in young people and women, completed suicides are three times as common in men and increase steadily with age. Because of the distress and stigma associated with suicide (attempted suicide has been punished as a crime in many societies and was illegal in the UK up till the 1960s) some have sought to show that almost all who commit suicide have some form of mental illness. This is fairly unconvincing but understandable as the state of mind of the person who committed suicide used to have serious implications (such as loss of the right to burial in consecrated ground).

The French sociologist Durkheim's book *La Suicide* published in 1897 opened a dramatically different perspective. It focused on the different rates of suicide in Catholics and Protestants and emphasized the importance of social isolation. He believed the Catholic faith protected from suicide and Catholic countries indeed do report lower suicide rates. This may be because they are more reluctant to acknowledge a death as suicide; in Dublin in the 1970s psychiatrists asked to assess the cause of sudden deaths concluded suicide four times as frequently as did local coroners. However there are undoubtedly variations in suicide rates between different countries.

Contrary to enduring myth, it is not Sweden that has the highest suicide rate but the countries of central and eastern Europe – e.g. Hungary, the Czech Republic, former East Germany. Currently there are astronomically high suicide rates in the collapsing former Soviet Union, with rates of 70 male suicides per 100,000 population (compared with the US 17 and the UK 12). Lithuania has the highest recorded rate at 76 per 100,000 and dramatically demonstrates the societal influence on suicide rates. As Russian speakers have gone from being the privileged elite to being the unwelcome minority their suicide rate is now much higher than Lithuanian speakers. It was previously the other way round. Nor are differences just reporting practices. The same national rankings are maintained in immigrants to the US from these different countries.

With such an environmental effect it could be argued that suicide is not a particularly psychiatric issue. But there is some encouragement that psychiatry is able to influence suicide. There is no specific 'anti-suicide treatment' (apart from some rather specialized psychological interventions to reduce suicidal ruminations in chronic depression). However, active identification of mental illnesses and their treatment may have an impact. There is no truth in the old wives' tale that those who talk about it don't do it (as 40 per cent consulting their GP in the preceding month testifies). A programme of teaching GPs on a Swedish island to enquire about depression and suicidal thinking and then treat the depression demonstrated a fall in the rate.

There are also known risk periods (e.g. just after discharge from psychiatric hospital) when extra support can make all the difference. The suicidal impulse is not static – it comes and goes. Consequently simply making it more difficult does reduce the risk – reducing the pack size of dangerous painkillers has significantly reduced deaths in the UK as has introducing non-lethal gas instead of the old coal-gas. Even netting off bridges helps – perhaps introducing delay and time to reflect, allowing the impulse to fade. The worldwide access to help lines such as the Samaritans who offer a sympathetic ear attests to the need to think things through and make human contact.

While the last century saw an overall decline in the suicide rate (with two marked dips during the wars) there is continuing cause for concern. There has been a steady rise, worldwide, in suicides in young men, and rates in some high-risk groups (small farmers, young South Asian women) are still distressingly high. Some of this is due to easy access to lethal means (pesticides and shotguns for farmers and an increasing use of car exhaust fumes) but some is probably due to weakening family ties, a sense of powerlessness plus the complications of drug and alcohol misuse.

Perhaps even more challenging is the change in society's attitudes towards suicide. While still desperately traumatic for the family it now attracts little stigma. Indeed it is increasingly seen as just one more option available to individuals with serious and painful illnesses (always a high-risk group) or those who feel their life has run its course. Switzerland has legalized assisted suicide in such cases, although those with mental illnesses are generally excluded. As living wills become increasingly accepted and if legally assisted suicide spreads from Switzerland (as it undoubtedly will), suicide may over time be seen as again more a moral and ethical issue of personal autonomy rather than a psychiatric one. Even more important, then, that suicide driven by judgements distorted through the lens of a mental illness should be prevented to protect such true autonomy.

Why is psychiatry a medical activity?

It is not accepted by everybody that mental health services should be run by psychiatrists (especially within the services themselves!). Are these 'mental health services' or 'psychiatric services'? Much of the controversy focuses on the 'medical model' which is thought to be too narrow and too dominant (Chapter 3). Psychology and social care can both make a strong case to offer the lead, and mental health nursing often stresses its independence. It will be obvious from what has been said so far that good practice (whether called mental health or psychiatric) requires a broader focus than just medicine. So how did psychiatry become so dominant?

One argument stems from the overlap between mental and physical diseases. Nearly all mental disease states can be mimicked by physical diseases and a failure to diagnose these may carry real risks. Thyroid disorders can present as depression ('myxoedema madness') or as an anxiety state. Deficiency of the B vitamin Niacin presents as dementia (Pellagra); myasthenia and early multiple sclerosis can easily be misdiagnosed as hysterical disorders. The list is extensive. This is, however, a pretty poor argument. Most patients come to mental health services via their family doctor who will filter out these physical problems. Where this doesn't happen it soon becomes clear that a patient is 'not like the other depressives' and a medical or neurological opinion easily sought. This may have been a more convincing argument when psychiatric patients were isolated away from other medical care in large mental hospitals but is hardly relevant in the 21st century.

A second argument is that many of the most successful treatments have been developed using a medical approach and, as many of these are drugs, you need a doctor to manage the treatment. The second part of this is not so convincing – psychiatrists attend and prescribe to residential facilities such as nursing homes and autism schools without being in charge. However, there is an argument that the 'medical model' has been very successful. By the medical model I mean an approach that, although drawing heavily on scientific theory and methods, is fundamentally pragmatic. If it works keep doing it; if it doesn't, stop it; if you're not sure conduct a careful experiment to find out. Psychiatry's overall independence from a defining theory, and its broadly scientific approach, are probably its major virtues. There is also within it a benign paternalism and willingness to accept responsibility that, while publicly decried, is often privately welcomed.

The status of doctors as the heads of mental hospitals arose, however, for quite other reasons. Certainly there was little doubt about the overlap between mental and physical disorders in the 19th century. Many mental hospital inpatients suffered from brain complications of syphilis that soon killed them and many more were severely physically ill. Doctors, however, did not *establish* mental hospitals but were put in charge of them (Chapter 2). This was not because they had effective treatments to offer but because their social standing and accountability made them effective guardians against abuse of patients. This abuse had been a widespread scandal throughout the madhouses the asylums replaced. At that time medical approaches to madness were probably more damaging than helpful. Doctors may have got their dominant position for surprising reasons but maintain it currently for more understandable ones. Whether they sustain it in the future is a different matter and will be returned to in Chapter 7.

A consultation with a psychiatrist

What will happen if your GP refers you to a psychiatrist? Practice varies but follows a broadly predictable pattern. It will almost certainly be an interview – most consultations are entirely conversational with no physical examinations or blood tests. It will usually last between 30 and 60 minutes.

The first thing the psychiatrist is likely to do is ask you to tell him or her in your own words what has been going on, what is distressing you, and what you think the problem is. Although the GP will have summarized this in the referral letter, most of us like to hear it from you and get a really clear picture. From then on the psychiatrist is likely to steer the discussion to get a broader picture of you and your life (your 'history'). He will find out about your upbringing and your family and usually ask detailed questions about family illnesses (especially psychiatric ones). After that he will ask about your health – both physical and psychiatric – over your lifetime and (particularly in younger people) about drug and alcohol use, as these often have a major impact on psychiatric problems. More detailed questioning is likely about areas relevant to your specific problem (important relationships, work stresses, etc.).

After taking a history the psychiatrist conducts what is called a 'mental state assessment'. This is a detailed evaluation of your symptoms – worries, mood, sleep, preoccupations. Usually this is also carried out as a conversation although sometimes there may be some quite formal questions and simple tests of memory. These are generally brief and not difficult – it's not like doing an IQ test.

After taking a history and conducting a mental state examination the psychiatrist will usually have come to an opinion of what the problem is (often called a 'formulation'). This formulation usually includes a diagnosis plus much more, such as thoughts about current difficulties and stresses that have brought on the problem. He will discuss these with you to get your opinion and then talk through the various options he thinks appropriate. This can involve a range of treatments (talking or tablets) or, rarely, a hospital admission. Surprisingly often, however, advice and reassurance is all that is needed. Nearly a quarter of referrals to psychiatrists in the UK are one-off consultations resulting in advice to the patient or GP.

Because so many psychiatric problems affect family members, psychiatrists will often want to talk with them, both to get a clearer understanding of what is going on but also to explain any proposed treatments to them (they may be very worried) and how best to help. Obviously this is not always appropriate – the circumstances may be very personal and private and adult patients have the right to total confidentiality if they wish it.

What the psychiatrist will *not* do is read your mind or ask trick questions. Sometimes it can seem this way because he appears to know much more than you've told him. There is nothing magical about this – it is simply that he will have heard similar stories before and will understand what is going on. That is, after all, his job – to know what depression and anxiety feel like and know how people cope with difficulties in their lives. Many find this, in itself, reassuring – that their problems are not unique; others have had similar difficulties and got over them. Similarly psychiatrists are not there to 'catch you out' with trick questions. They want to know what you are going through and give advice on how to manage it. What will also not happen is a sudden admission to hospital against your will. There are no psychiatric diagnoses that require immediate compulsory hospitalization. That only happens when there is overwhelming evidence of real risk and usually after much discussion and with a lot of involvement of family and GP.

Having made his assessment and discussed the treatment with you he may make a further appointment either for you to see him or another member of the team for treatment (e.g. a nurse or psychologist) or say that you don't need to come back. Whichever happens he will write to your GP and keep him informed.

So we now know a bit about the scope of psychiatry – how it fits into the other approaches to understanding the mind, what sort of disorders or illnesses it treats, and the major treatment approaches. You may by now regret having started reading – so many uncertainties, overlaps, and contradictions. Couldn't it have been simpler? Well probably not. If we were to invent psychiatry from scratch it would be different. What we have, however, developed piecemeal over the last two centuries. It is the product of powerful competing forces and momentous historical developments and is confronted just now by truly remarkable advances in the neurosciences. So keep reading and by the end it should make some sort of sense – you will remember that you were never promised certainty.

Chapter 2
Asylums and the origins of psychiatry

Psychiatry's history is manageably short – barely 200 years. The mentally deranged have always been recognized and where they could not be cared for within the family some makeshift provision was made – private madhouses and spas for the rich and workhouses for the poor. Workhouses contained everyone who could not care for themselves – the feeble-minded, the sick, the feckless, and the unemployed. Conditions were grim (deliberately so to discourage the burden on the public purse) and the mentally ill often fared badly from other inmates who were impatient with them or took advantage of them. Private madhouses were hardly that much better. There was no training required to own or run them. Their main purpose seemed to be to hide mad members of rich families from view, either to protect the family's reputation or to appropriate their fortunes. The harsh treatment of the much loved King George III generated powerful antipathy towards them in late 18th-century England.

Bedlam was the first major public madhouse, opened in London in 1685 and still in existence as the much-reformed Bethlem Royal Hospital. The exhibition of the inmates was a popular public pastime in the early 18th century and generated revulsion in more educated quarters. France had established its Hotel Dieu and Hôpital Général in 1656 (the Bicêtre for men and Salpêtrière for women) which, despite their names, were not hospitals, but general establishments for custodial care more akin to workhouses. Tollhäuser (fools' houses) had been established in medieval Europe. The first US insane ward was established in a Boston Almshouse in 1729 and the first US Psychiatric Hospital in 1773 in Williamsburg, Virginia.

The York retreat

The impetus to separate the mentally ill and provide more appropriate care came not from doctors but from social reformers and reflected an emerging concern with the dignity of man. In our risk-obsessed days it is sobering to realize that asylums were proposed more to protect the deranged individual from society than vice versa. In France in 1792, Pinel dramatically and symbolically removed the chains from inmates in the Bicêtre and in England a Quaker family, the Tukes, proposed and built the first Asylum in York. The Tukes were convinced by the writings of Pinel and Esquirol that a calm and harmonious environment, close to nature and with kindness and predictable routines ('moral therapy'), would bring peace to a troubled mind. The York retreat was built to contain 30 patients; opened in 1796 it achieved remarkable results – many early patients were discharged home improved or even cured. It attracted attention from all over the world and visitors came from the US and throughout Europe to study and replicate it. The UK developed early a liberal regime, reluctant to use mechanical restraints such as chains or belts (later championed by John Conolly in the 'non-restraint movement').

The asylum movement

In the 1820s the asylum movement began and over the next 70 years hundreds were built for the reception of indigent 'lunatics' in each county in England, in most European countries, and across America. The scale of investment is hard to conceive of now, with enormous, well appointed buildings to house

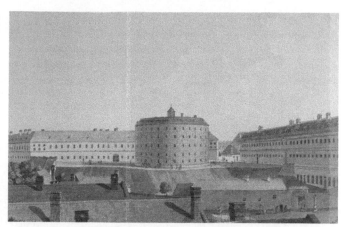

1. Narrenturm ('Fools' Tower') situated alongside the Vienna General Hospital, the first modern general hospital in Europe, built by Emperor Joseph II in 1787

several hundred patients each. The physical conditions within the asylum (space, heating, food, recreation) would have been significantly better than most patients could have expected at home with their families. The principles of moral therapy dictated that asylums should be spacious, away from busy towns, placed in the countryside with extensive grounds. High airy locations were selected because of current theories implicating mists and 'miasmas' in disease.

Doctors were put in charge of asylums primarily because they were easy to hold accountable to the board of governors. There were few effective medical interventions and the medical superintendent's role was predominantly administrative and disciplinary. He didn't even have the power to admit or discharge patients – that was usually held by the local magistrates.

Asylums started well, often admitting recent cases – many of whom recovered. They soon seized up, however, with those who did not recover and so became overcrowded. Throughout the latter part of the 19th century and early 20th century, the recovery rate in mental hospitals declined steadily because of an increasing concentration of these more severe cases. Therapeutic optimism gradually faded and conditions (though still much better than the workhouse) deteriorated.

Throughout the 19th century investment in asylums was maintained. They were kept high on the agenda in the US by the influential social reformer Dorothea Dix and the physician Benjamin Rush and in England by strong central support from the influential social reformer Lord Shaftsbury. Initially quite small institutions, they rapidly grew to several hundred inmates each in Europe and up to several thousand in the US, where the building programme started a bit later and continued longer. Between 1903 and 1933 the number of patients in US mental hospitals more than doubled from 143,000 to 366,000. Most of these were in institutions of more than 1,000 beds and US mental hospitals continued to expand. The largest was the Georgia State Sanatorium at Milledgeville which by 1950 housed over 10,000 patients.

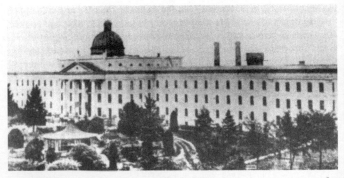

2. Georgia state sanatorium at Milledgeville: the largest state mental hospital in the USA. At its height in 1950 it housed over 10,000 patients

The non-restraint movement

Cultural values are strongly reflected in the care of the mentally ill.
This is still the case despite the globalization of mental health
research. At the start of the asylum movement the UK and US
focused on human rights and, particularly in the UK, on treating
patients with as little physical restriction as possible. John Conolly,
the physician superintendent at Hanwell Asylum, became the
leading proponent of managing patients without strait-jackets or
chains. He emphasized the value of well trained and unflappable
staff and used isolation to allow patients to calm down. A US visitor
to Conolly commented that English patients must be more
tractable and that the approach would 'never work at home'. This
tradition has continued and the UK became the first country to run
some mental hospitals entirely without locked doors (Dingleton in
Scotland was a fully 'open-door' hospital by 1948 – *before* the new
drugs, see Chapter 3). The UK approach remains unusual in its
total absence of mechanical restraints to control agitated patients.
Whether its reliance on medication to achieve this is always a good
thing is, of course, open to question.

Psychiatry as a profession

Medical superintendents were responsible for running the
asylums – ensuring there was enough food, sacking drunken staff,
preventing abuse, and proposing discharge to the board if
patients recovered. Some of the more able (such as John
Conolly) became highly skilled in man-management and also
took a leading role in the design of new asylums. The early
asylum movement produced some remarkable architectural
achievements but relatively few therapeutic ones. There was no
specific training to be an asylum doctor – you went there and
worked alongside the superintendent and if you were lucky
you eventually replaced him. These were, however, generally
thoughtful men (they were all men) and interested in science.
In the 1840s they founded their own professional bodies –

the Association of Medical Superintendents in the UK in 1841
(later to become, 1865, the Royal Medical Psychological Society
and in 1971 the Royal College of Psychiatrists). The formation of
this professional association in 1841 coincided with the naming
of the dinosaur – a coincidence not lost on the profession's
detractors.

'Germany' – psychiatry's birthplace

In the second half of the 19th century there was a remarkable
intellectual flourishing in German-speaking Europe. The
collection of states that came to make up modern Germany were
rivals of each other and characterized by local centres of
government with prestigious universities and institutions. Unlike
France at the time (where everything happened in Paris) there
were several culturally and linguistically linked, but independent,
centres of innovation – Munich, Berlin, Vienna, Zurich. From
these came the great founding fathers of modern psychiatry:
Griesinger, Morel, Alzheimer, Kraepelin, Bleuler, Freud, Jung.
The first professor of psychiatry was established in Berlin
(Griesinger 1864) and there were six by 1882. Compare this to
England where the first professor of psychiatry was appointed in
1948.

These academic posts were not, on the whole, placed in mental
hospitals nor were they dedicated to the treatment of the legions
of psychotic and demented patients who inhabited them. Most
research was conducted in university clinics and most was
focused on detailed examinations of the nervous system in an
attempt to elucidate the mechanisms of the 'degeneration' that
was thought to underlie mental illnesses. Three of the most
influential figures found their way into the area for more personal
reasons. Falling in love was the reason for both Kraepelin and
Freud and family concern for Bleuler. Freud and Kraepelin had
successful research posts in university departments (Freud was
dissecting the nervous system of eels). A research career at that

time was incompatible (in terms of both income and time) with marriage and a family. However, both had met the women they wanted to marry so there was no alternative but to relinquish their promising research posts and look for a 'real' job. Luckily we know that both had long and happy marriages. Bleuler was born and brought up in the Zurich cantonment and didn't want to move. His sister suffered from schizophrenia and he was close to her and it seemed logical to return to a job at the Burghölzi hospital where she was cared for. These three men moulded modern psychiatry.

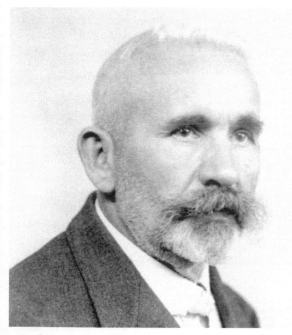

3. Emil Kraepelin (1856–1926): distinguished dementia praecox (later called schizophrenia) from manic depressive disorder and laid the foundation for a rational classification of psychiatric disorders

Kraepelin (1856–1926)

Kraepelin moved with his new wife in 1886 to become an asylum doctor in Dorpat in what is now Estonia. The professional classes spoke German but his patients didn't – consequently he didn't understand a word they said and could not usefully interview them. What he did do was study their case notes and observe the fluctuations in their illnesses. From this he made the distinction between schizophrenia (which he called 'dementia praecox' meaning early dementia) and manic depressive disorder. Although in their acute phases it was difficult to distinguish the two disorders, important differences emerged over time. The dementia praecox patients never (he believed) fully recovered and with each bout of acute illness became more disabled. Based on the course of the illnesses he established the classification into the two major functional psychoses that persists to this day.

'Kraeplinian' implies a pessimistic view of schizophrenia (if defined by its poor outcome it can only be diagnosed if there *is* a poor outcome) and of exaggerating its difference from manic depressive disorder. However demonstrating that you could successfully classify the psychoses at all brought enormous benefits. Once you can distinguish different groups you can begin to make sensible predictions about outcome ('prognosis') and develop a clearer picture of each illness. Having distinguished these two it allowed psychiatrists to start distinguishing the others (dementia, cerebral syphilis, intoxications). At the simplest level it gave psychiatry a reason to pay more attention to patients' illnesses and provided a basis for some rudimentary predictions and development of treatments.

Kraepelin became a celebrated and influential figure who travelled widely in his own lifetime. He was a passionate advocate for the temperance movement and on a lecture tour of Italy it was not so much his radical diagnostic ideas that amazed his Italian colleagues as the fact that he refused to drink wine. Indeed, he

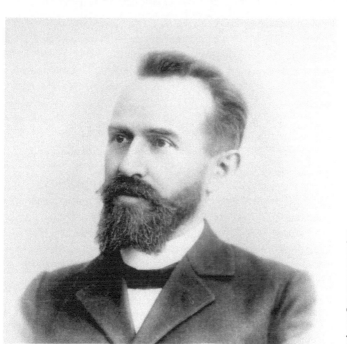

4. Eugen Bleuler (1857–1939): first used the term 'schizophrenia', in 1911

considered his campaign against alcohol his main contribution to humanity.

Eugen Bleuler (1857–1939)

Bleuler first coined the term schizophrenia in 1911. It followed many years of careful study in the Burghölzi hospital in Zurich. Bleuler's situation could hardly have been more different from Kraepelin's. He had grown up using the same dialect as his patients, lived in the hospital where his sister was a patient with schizophrenia, and often spent evenings talking to his patients. In every way he was primed to try to understand and make sense of their inner world rather than just observe as Kraepelin had done.

His definition of schizophrenia is based on the content of the patient's experience. This approach allowed him to make the diagnosis (providing the features were present) even if the outcome was good. Of course there were many schizophrenia patients with poor outcomes but Bleuler confirmed there were some with good outcomes.

Bleuler considered that the primary disturbances in schizophrenia were a withdrawal from close relationships and disturbances of thinking and mood. He believed that hallucinations and delusions were attempts by the patient to make sense of these experiences. He defined schizophrenia using his famous 'Four As' – *Autism* (withdrawal), *Affect* (mood disturbances), *Association* (thought disorder – different associations or meanings being attached to words), *Ambivalence* (lack of direction and motivation). Bleuler's approach has been superseded in recent years by a focus on the 'positive' symptoms (delusions, hallucinations, thought disorder) because of their greater ease of recognition and responsiveness to drug treatment. His was certainly a more humane approach to this, the most devastating of the mental illnesses, which accords meaning to the experiences of even the most deteriorated patient.

Sigmund Freud (1856–1939)

Like Kraepelin Freud had to abandon his preferred career for marriage. He pursued the only available alternative for a Jewish doctor at that time – private practice. Freud had little experience of asylums and worked almost exclusively with neurotic patients; he always recognized the limitations of his approaches for more severely ill patients. However, a careful reading of his case histories leaves little doubt that he treated some pretty disturbed individuals. His investigations took him in a completely different direction: the founding of psychoanalysis (Chapter 3). He thought of himself as much a scientist exploring the mind as a doctor curing it. He always believed that physical treatments (medicines) would eventually be the cure for mental illnesses.

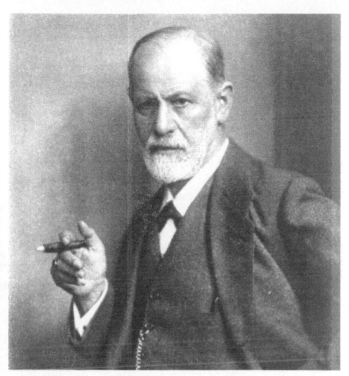

5. Freud (1856–1939): the father of psychoanalysis

We might anticipate antagonism or avoidance between these groups a century ago but this doesn't appear to have been the case. This was still a 'pre medical-model' psychiatry. Working in large asylums, all that was available to the doctors after they had classified their patients into broad diagnostic groups was to talk with them. Moral therapy evolved into a rough and ready psychotherapy. Few believed this cured the disease, but the role of doctors has never been restricted to just cure, but also to bringing relief from suffering. The journals of asylum doctors of this time testify to the time spent talking with patients – attempting to bring comfort and using reasoning to calm them.

The work of another great German psychiatrist, Karl Jaspers (1883–1969), exemplifies this. Jaspers wrote his masterpiece in Heidelberg by the age of 30: *General Psychopathology* (1913). This book is still in print and has never been bettered as a description of the mental processes in psychotic illnesses. Jaspers was initially quite comfortable with the writings of the psychoanalysts and his book clearly distinguishes the two different approaches to researching mental illnesses. The first is *verstehen* 'understanding' and the second *erklären* 'explaining'. Both were considered legitimate and necessary: what is the meaning of what the patient says and what is causing it? This is a dichotomy that still causes conflict in psychiatry – particularly between the psychologically minded and the biologically minded. Jaspers eventually lost patience with Freud because he felt that he implied that to understand was to explain. In its origins psychiatry needed and valued both approaches.

The first medical model

The end of the asylum era (Chapter 3) was foreshadowed by the 'first medical model' in the 1920s and 1930s. Interest in psychiatry had received a boost during the First World War with the need to treat shell-shocked soldiers, while at the same time the asylums had become even more overcrowded and neglected. It was only from the 1920s onwards that really effective treatments were discovered and introduced. These caused widespread changes in attitudes and restored optimism. 'Lunatic' was replaced with 'mental patient', 'asylum' with 'mental hospital', 'certification' with 'involuntary admission', and voluntary admissions became common for the first time: a truly revolutionary change in perspective.

There had been a steady improvement in the drugs used to control agitation prior to this time but two new treatments were epoch making – malaria treatment for cerebral syphilis and electro-convulsive therapy.

Julius Wagner-Jauregg (1857–1940) and malaria treatment

Wagner-Jauregg was the only psychiatrist to be awarded the Nobel Prize for Medicine before Sigmund Freud in 1939. He received it for his 1917 introduction of malaria treatment for cerebral syphilis (then called general paralysis of the insane, GPI). Before effective treatments for syphilis, a small proportion of chronically infected patients went on to develop the disease in the brain with disastrous consequences. It often took 20 years to develop, by which time the patient might be a settled family man. The terror it represented for 19th-century society is vividly captured in Ibsen's play *Ghosts*. Onset of mental symptoms was sudden and dramatic. The philosopher Nietzsche inexplicably embraced a horse that was being abused in the street in Turin and within days was confined to a mental hospital; he died 11 years later never having recovered. Deterioration was tragic and humiliating. It was often associated with delusions of grandeur (hence all those cartoons of patients convinced they were Napoleon), and ended in dementia.

Wagner-Jauregg's treatment consisted of infecting the patient with malaria parasites and waiting, with careful nursing, while the high fever raged. Over 10–12 cycles this killed the syphilis germs. The malaria could afterwards be treated with quinine. This treatment was difficult and risky but the alternative held no hope. GPI was effectively cleared from mental hospitals long before effective antibiotics arrived. Malaria treatment restored optimism to mental hospitals and strengthened the professional pride of the doctors and nurses who had to manage this difficult, but effective, treatment. It also forged clearer links with general hospitals where the patients often had to go to be treated. In doing this it became clear that involuntary patients would often cooperate with treatment and this stimulated a reassessment of the need for so much compulsion.

Electro-convulsive therapy

While malaria treatment is purely of historical interest, electro-convulsive therapy (ECT) is still widely used. Psychiatrists knew that epileptic seizures often caused profound changes in mood – either exciting or calming patients in the hours after a fit. It was also thought that epilepsy was uncommon in patients with schizophrenia so the idea developed that perhaps fits protected patients against this disease. Fits were induced in schizophrenia patients from 1935 by getting them to inhale camphor or by injecting a chemical called metrazol. The results were promising, with many patients improving. Unfortunately the experience (in particular the minutes leading up to the fit after the metrazol was injected) were very unpleasant indeed, with mounting dread, so many patients refused the treatments.

An Italian, Cerletti, came up with the idea of using a weak electric current to initiate the fit and used it on his first patient in 1938 with striking results. Several psychiatrists started to use ECT and its results were truly remarkable. While it did calm very agitated schizophrenic patients, its most dramatic results were with depressed patients, many of whom made sustained recoveries. If this all sounds a bit barbaric it pays to remember that depressed patients in the 1930s (even in very good mental hospitals) often stayed for years and up to one fifth *died* during the admission.

Initially ECT was given without anaesthetic and clearly was a frightening experience often with complications of small fractures if the fit was very strong, headache, and memory loss. For the last 50 years patients have received a short-acting anaesthetic and a chemical to block the muscle contractions so there is no fit to see and no risk of fractures. Headache and memory loss are still problems but patients don't recall the actual seizure.

The discovery and durability of ECT is typical of many developments in psychiatry. The idea that started it (that epilepsy protected against schizophrenia) was wrong but the treatment worked, although more in depression than schizophrenia. We still don't know why it works, but it certainly does. It remains one of the most effective treatments in psychiatry and (despite its wider reputation) the one that most patients who have had it say they would want again.

Mental health legislation

Psychiatry is unique within medicine in being able to compel treatment against a patient's clearly expressed wishes. Consequently most countries have evolved specific legislation to permit this and to monitor it. The whole of the asylum movement was firmly based in such legislation. The developments in England in the 19th century are easy to follow because it was an early nation-state with centralized government and little scope for regional variation.

The first legislation was to regulate madhouses. All this did was to register them. It set no standards but could close an individual madhouse in the event of flagrant abuse. The purpose of the Asylum Act of 1808 and the Lunacy Act of 1845 was to ensure that care was provided and prevent exploitation of the vulnerable mentally ill. It allowed for 'the removal of the furiously mad' from workhouses to the asylum.

Over the next half century, public concerns shifted from the neglect and abuse of the indigent mentally ill to the spectre of malevolent incarceration of the sane to rob them of their wealth. The 'Alleged Lunatics' Friends Society', with an admiral of the fleet as chairman, gained considerable parliamentary and public support in late 19th-century Britain. Georgina Weldon (a 'spirited, attractive, wealthy and well connected woman') filled the Covent Garden Opera House in London in 1883 for a rally to challenge her recent incarcerations, and eventually won her case. Increasing public disquiet was reflected in the 1890 Lunacy Act. This highly legalistic document, several hundred pages and 342 sections long, prioritized the protection of patients' rights to such an extent that early and voluntary treatment became virtually impossible. The leading historian of mental health legislation, Kathleen Jones, wrote that 'it stopped progress in mental health policy in its tracks for half a century'.

So swings the pendulum of public attitudes to mental health. Virtually every developed land is struggling to balance legal rights and therapeutic needs, to balance society's needs with the patient's. We will return to this in Chapter 6 but it is sobering to be reminded that we have been here before.

Asylums limped onwards for another 50–60 years, mired in legislation and inhibited from innovation apart from the welcome treatment advances in the 1920s and 1930s. It was to be another 30 years before this awesome international institution was finally challenged and moved towards its end. This is the subject of Chapter 3.

Chapter 3
The move into the community

After decades of being hidden from view, the mentally ill are now very much in the public eye. Hardly a week goes by without some headline about the plight of the homeless mentally ill or an incident involving a disturbed individual. 'Care in the Community' has become an international preoccupation with much soul-searching and fear of violence and disorder. How has this situation come about? Is it really so disastrous and, if so, what can be done about it?

Deinstitutionalization

The number of psychiatric beds in the West has shrunk to less than a third of what it was in 1955. Nearly every large mental hospital in the UK and most in the US have closed. The few remaining house only a fraction of the patients they once did. Chronic wards where long-stay patients lived out their lives have virtually disappeared. In the mid-1950s there were 500,000 psychiatric inpatients in the USA and 160,000 in the UK. Now there are less than 100,000 in the USA and less than 30,000 in the UK. This trend is virtually worldwide. This process, inelegantly entitled 'deinstitutionalization' started by reducing overcrowding and then closing wards. The last 15 years has finally seen the closure of whole mental hospitals.

It is usual to attribute this emptying of the asylums to the

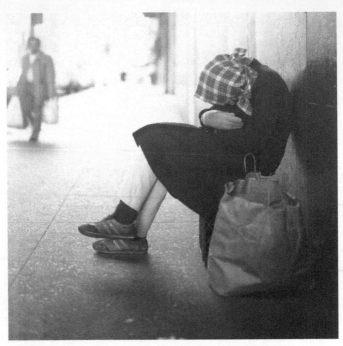

6. A 'bag lady': a homeless, mentally ill woman with her few possessions – an increasingly common sight in cities throughout the world during the 1990s and often blamed on the rapid closure of mental hospitals

discovery of antipsychotic drugs in the early 1950s. This was clearly the major force but it is not the whole story. Fundamental changes in social attitudes towards the mentally ill were afoot before these drugs were introduced. The impact of the new drugs varied enormously – from wholesale discharges in some countries, to almost no effect in others. Social attitudes and radical rethinking within psychiatry also exerted powerful influences. Later, financial considerations entered the picture. But let us start with the drugs.

The drug revolution

Like so many important discoveries chlorpromazine's antipsychotic effect was found by pure chance. A French navy anaesthetist researching trauma and shock noted how it calmed patients post-operatively without sedating them. Two psychiatrists, Delay and Deneke, tried the drug in St Anne's hospital in Paris in 1952 and were astounded by the results. By the tenth patient they knew they had a breakthrough. Over the next four years chlorpromazine became the front-line treatment in psychotic illnesses and the atmosphere in psychiatric wards was totally transformed.

At its most immediate the drugs humanized the wards. Staff could begin to get to know their patients rather than just controlling them. Episodes of illness were both shorter and less disturbed so that rehabilitation and early discharge (before family relationships and jobs were lost for good) became realistic possibilities. Initially the drugs were used only for treating acute episodes but by the 1970s it was realized that staying on them reduced the risk of further breakdowns. This 'maintenance therapy' has become the cornerstone of long-term treatment of schizophrenia and other psychoses.

Over the last 50 years a whole range of antipsychotics has been developed. Most are about equally effective but their side effects are very different. The original chlorpromazine-like drugs often made patients stiff and lethargic. Newer drugs avoid the stiffness but can cause weight gain and diabetes. Some of these drugs became available as long-acting injections which means the patient can forget about taking them as long as they get their injection every two to four weeks.

The drug revolution was not restricted to antipsychotics. The first of the antidepressants (imipramine) was introduced in 1958. These had a longer lasting effect than ECT and were more acceptable to many more patients – by the early 1980s US physicians were writing 10 million antidepressant prescriptions a year. Lithium carbonate (a naturally occurring substance) was noted in 1949 to have a calming effect. It was introduced as a long-term 'mood-stabilizing' treatment for manic depressive disorder in 1968 and has substantially reduced the risk of further breakdowns.

This is not the place to detail the developments in modern psychiatric drugs but just to note that the progress has been accelerating. We now have a wide range of drugs for most recognized disorders. However, these are not 'magic bullets'. No drug will completely cure all patients with a specific disorder but, carefully chosen, drug treatments can make a real difference to the vast majority of patients with mental illnesses. The very success of these newer drugs poses risks for overuse and ethical dilemmas which will be picked up in Chapter 6.

The revolution in social attitudes
The Second World War

Psychiatry changed radically during the Second World War and gained new confidence because its contribution was highly valued (both in the selection of soldiers and in the acute treatment of combat disorders). Its increased profile and importance brought many doctors into it who would never have contemplated work in asylums. Fresh minds were brought to old problems. Previously healthy men transformed into nervous wrecks by battle challenged old fatalistic genetic hypotheses. Dramatic recoveries from battle-trauma with practical treatments (e.g. barbiturate injections to release or 'abreact' emotions from recent terrifying experiences) confirmed the role of stress and trauma. Psychiatry became an active and optimistic, almost glamorous, branch of medicine.

Therapeutic communities

The treatment of acute war neuroses by drug treatments was not the only Second World War advance. Psychiatrists with a psychoanalytical training obtained influential military adviser posts in both the US and UK. They explored how organizations themselves could influence mental health and recovery and developed the 'therapeutic community'.

The therapeutic community emphasized that the *organization* of hospitals (or prisons or schools or offices for that matter) has a major impact on the well-being of those in them. For psychiatric patients it can be an opportunity for self-learning and recovery. Army psychiatrists noted the problems of treating ordinary private soldiers for psychological problems because they, the doctors, were senior officers. Rank and status simply got in the way. They actively reduced status differences in their units, encouraging informality and stressing the patients' capacity to work together to help each other and solve problems. This allowed neurotic and disabled individuals to learn new ways of dealing with their problems in a democratic, tolerant, and enquiring group environment.

The therapeutic community movement improved care in mental hospitals and subsequently in prisons and residential schools for disturbed children and adolescents. It is a victim of its own success, as its lessons have become so accepted (even in commercial organizations) that their origins are forgotten. Psychoanalysis has suffered a similar fate.

'Institutional neurosis' and 'total institutions'

About the same time it was recognized that traditional mental hospital environments could have a profoundly damaging impact on patients. Hospitals could themselves be the *cause* of some of the problems that they were striving to treat. Long-stay patients (usually those suffering from schizophrenia) who had been inpatients for years or decades, were noted to be apathetic, self-neglecting, and isolated. This had always been considered a consequence of schizophrenia (a so-called 'schizophrenia defect state') and the plight and dependency of these individuals was one of the arguments sustaining mental hospitals.

This aspect of schizophrenia (unlike the acute symptoms of hallucinations, delusions, and agitation) did not respond much to the new drugs. But the hospital itself appeared to make a difference. It had always been known that there were good mental hospitals and bad ones. A study of three hospitals of similar size and staffing with equally ill schizophrenia patients in the 1960s found markedly different levels of apathy and self-neglect. The study showed that the differences related to the levels of activity and variety provided in daily routines.

A psychiatrist, Russell Barton, went further and proposed that much of this apathy was a response to living in an institution which denied personal responsibility. The apathy was a consequence of disuse – you simply stopped looking after yourself because somebody else always did it for you. Barton called this 'institutional neurosis' to stress that its cause was the hospital, not the schizophrenia. He reorganized things to give his patients more independence, with remarkable results. Many patients flourished in the new regime and were soon discharged. Rehabilitation (helping patients regain their lost skills and abilities) became a preoccupation in most mental hospitals and optimism grew that most of these apathetic, disabled patients would no longer need inpatient care.

'Institutional neurosis' stimulated change but its extent was undoubtedly exaggerated. There *is* an apathetic state that develops as part of long-term schizophrenia but it had been magnified by hospital routines. There were even some patients who had recovered and the staff had simply not noticed! Many of Barton's early patients embraced their independence effortlessly, but such 'overlooked' patients are now rare and ongoing support is usually needed.

Erving Goffman and total institutions

The Three Hospitals Study and Russell Barton's institutional neurosis shook up the professions but they pale alongside the international shock wave caused by *Asylums* (1961) – a book by the American sociologist Erving Goffman. This groundbreaking study (he worked 'undercover' for a year as a cleaner in the wards of an enormous mental hospital in Washington, DC), his clear and radical thinking and, not least, his elegant writing simply stunned the establishment. Goffman described in convincing detail what *really* went on in an asylum – not what people *thought* went on. Doctors and nurses thought they shared a common understanding but Goffman showed that they did not – doctors judged patients using a disease and treatment model, whereas the nurses made judgements based more on behaviour and on patient motives. More tellingly doctors thought they ran the units but it was clear that for day-to-day life nurses, aides (and even other patients) set the rules and culture and held the authority. Goffman was not sympathetic to the asylum.

He went further. He concluded that the dehumanizing and degradation of patients resulting from inflexible routines and the absence of individualized care were not simply the regrettable effects of poorly trained staff and lack of resources (the usual explanations). He argued that such institutions *actively* eroded individuality. This was particularly characteristic of what he called 'total institutions' such as asylums, prisons, and the army. These typically meet all their Members' needs – e.g. food, shelter, company, leisure. They rely on rigid distinctions between staff and patients (or prisoners and warders, or officers and men) and on demeaning rituals to erode and suppress individual identity. He argued that they do this to enforce discipline and make large groups of people more easily manageable. In the hospital in which he worked he cited the highly structured admission process that included not only medical examination but delousing, bathing, and hair cutting for all patients as one such potent and symbolic degradation.

Whilst (understandably) initially unwelcome to the professions Goffman's writings have been a major force in driving the closure of the mental hospitals. His book *Asylums* is still *the* most quoted text in modern sociology 40 years after its publication. Ken Kesey's 1962 book *One Flew Over the Cuckoo's Nest* (and its enormously successful film adaptation staring Jack Nicholson in 1975) vividly portrayed the unacceptable face of such large impersonal asylums.

The rights and abuse of the mentally ill

I have focused so far on the forces from within the professions that led to deinstitutionalization. However, just as with the origins of the asylums (Chapter 2), the social climate of the time was probably as influential, if not more so. Directly after the Second World War Europe burned with a spirit of change and a thirst for social justice. The old order was in disgrace and the rights of the common man were the priority of both returning soldiers and returned governments. Democracy and social inclusion (though not called

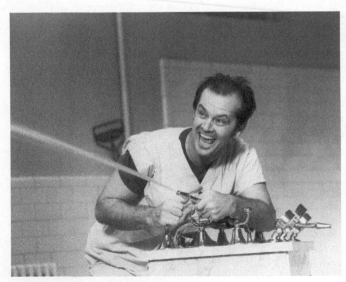

7. *One Flew Over the Cuckoo's Nest*: Jack Nicholson as the rebellious Randle McMurphy in Milos Forman's 1975 film depicting a repressive mental hospital

that then) dominated the international agenda, whether in education, health, or housing. The rights of disadvantaged groups to take full part in this new society were strongly defended and the mentally ill were one such group. Their wholesale liquidation in Nazi Germany only served to underline their rights for protection. Nowhere is this so clearly demonstrated as in changes in Mental Health Law. In the UK, for example, the 1890 Lunacy Act focused on protecting the rights of the sane not to be judged insane (with scant regard to the rights or welfare of the insane) whereas the 1959 Mental Health Act focused on protecting the rights of the mentally ill by ensuring due process and review of their care and detention.

A series of scandals about the abuse of mental patients surfaced in the 1960s and 1970s. Revelation after revelation of degrading and inadequate care followed inquiries into several mental hospitals. The reports ranged from the denial of dignity through to frank abuse and assault. These scandals painted a recurrent picture of large isolated institutions (size appears crucial, with risk escalating rapidly above about 400 patients), with a poorly trained but very cohesive staff group, many of whom had followed their parents into the job. The practices Goffman had identified were very much in evidence, with little attention to individualized treatment or care.

These revelations produced understandable revulsion and strengthened resolve to reform or remove asylums. In 1960 the UK Health Minister prophesied their demise but predicted that professional attitudes would outlive the bricks and mortar. The Italian reforms drove this home. Their charismatic originator, the psychiatrist and philosopher Franco Bassaglia, believed that the mental hospital was fundamentally unreformable (see Chapter 5) and abolition was the only way forward. Law 180 in 1978 prohibited compulsory admissions to mental hospitals immediately and demanded their total closure within three years.

At this time the whole legitimacy of psychiatry was being called into question. The anti-psychiatry movement (Chapter 5) led by R. D. Laing, Thomas Szasz, and Michel Foucault had been borne aloft in the student revolts of 1968. Their books became campus bibles of the 1970s across the whole of Europe and the US.

By the early 1980s the downsizing and closing of mental hospitals was an established international movement led and articulated by mental health professionals, mainly psychiatrists. However, despite smaller numbers of inpatients, the cost of mental health care *increased* as staffing standards came more in line with those in general medicine and as decades of neglect were addressed. The financial advantages of closing whole mental hospitals became obvious to governments who have driven this agenda for the last 20 years (often now *opposed* by the professionals). It is this 'unholy alliance between therapeutic liberals and fiscal conservatives' as one astute US observer noted which has driven deinstitutionalization over the last 30 years.

'Transinstitutionalization' and 'reinstitutionalization'

When the asylums were built they did not take their first new patients from family homes but from prisons and workhouses. One worrying aspect of deinstitutionalization is that some of the reduction means more mentally ill patients are transferred back to prisons. As psychiatric units became smaller and more therapeutic in orientation, many of their more difficult patients (who previously would have remained for longer periods on locked wards) were denied access and ended up in prison. This regrettable trend has been exacerbated in parts of the world where the criteria for compulsory care have been so tightened that they require evidence of immediate danger. California now has more psychotic individuals in prison than in mental hospitals.

So the rate of deinstitutionalization is not quite so dramatic as hospital closures might suggest. Indeed, in the last five years or so, the signs are of a slight reverse, with more mentally ill people in some form of supervised accommodation. There are many factors involved (see below) but one is undoubtedly increasing intolerance of risk.

Care in the community

'Any fool can close a mental hospital' remarked a senior UK health official in the 1980s. He quickly added that the skill was not in closing the hospital but providing alternative care. Recognizable forms of modern community care have been developing since the 1930s – psychiatric day hospitals in Russia, outpatient departments in both the US and the UK, mobile clinics in the Netherlands. However from the 1960s onwards real effort went into community services as an *alternative* to mental hospitals rather than simply as a complement.

District general hospital units and day hospitals

The building of small inpatient units either in or alongside local general hospitals stood for the destigmatizing of the mentally ill and the move away from the mental hospital. These units were small, usually 40–100 beds. They catered for acute, short-term patients and could usually rely on the mental hospital for back up. They are an international phenomenon but practice reflects local customs. In the US they embody a strong tradition of general hospital liaison psychiatry; in Germany an academic psychosomatic tradition of psychotherapeutic treatment of physical illnesses; in the UK a mental hospital tradition adapted to more rapid discharge. The Italian reforms insisted on a complete break, substituting tiny, very short-term admission units.

It is sobering to reflect, however, that in the new expanded Europe over half of psychiatric inpatients are still cared for in traditional mental hospitals with little, if any, real community provision. US practice varies enormously between states, from highly community-based services to extensive reliance on old mental hospitals. Locating psychiatric units in general hospitals and keeping them small guards against many of the problems of asylums, but they have their own problems, such as being cramped and less tolerant. They may also have difficulties with very difficult patients and usually cannot offer the breadth of activities and treatments of larger units. They are, however, a first essential step out from the asylum into the community.

Community mental health teams (CMHTs) and community mental health centres (CMHCs)

Breaking the dominance of mental hospitals involved moving services closer to patients. Services needed to be accessible and not too frightening so that patients and families would approach them early for help. 'Sector psychiatry' arose to meet the challenge. Asylums took all the patients from a defined catchment area (often a whole county or a city). The sector approach divided this into small manageable areas (40,000–100,000 population) to provide easily accessible, fairly comprehensive care.

France and the UK led the way in this development. The French 'secteur' arose from sociological theory and emphasized crisis intervention. The service was restricted to psychotic patients and remains patchy. The UK approach was more comprehensive but entirely pragmatic, much less theoretical. Local care followed 1950s legislation requiring compulsory detained patients to be offered outpatient follow-up and requiring the involvement of social services. Collaboration was not feasible from distant mental hospitals; linking with social workers and family doctors was only realistic in small neighbourhoods. The sector approach meant psychiatrists and nurses and social workers started working together in teams.

In the UK this development was made possible by 'community psychiatric nurses' (CPNs). These are nurses who work almost exclusively outside hospital, most often visiting psychotic patients in their homes to ensure they carry on with their medicine but also helping to solve day-to-day practical problems. Starting from two in 1953 there are now more CPNs than psychiatrists in the UK. CPNs and psychiatrists working together established multidisciplinary team practice, gradually incorporating social workers, clinical psychologists, and occupational therapists.

Community mental health teams assess the broad range of mental health problems (from depression to psychosis) and offer treatment in clinics, patients' homes, day hospitals, and (when needed) as inpatients. They have become the norm throughout Europe and many parts of the world. The Italian reforms most clearly encapsulated this model of care, emphasizing informality, local knowledge, and flexible access.

Most CMHTs are broadly similar. In Italy and the UK the same team usually looks after patients both in and out of the hospital, but in much of Europe and the US these responsibilities are separate. In some services CMHTs see the whole range of mental health problems; in others they may restrict themselves to severe psychoses. There has been a recent move to replace CMHTs with a range of specialized teams (e.g. for crisis, for long-term support, for first onset patients). While the focus of these teams differs, their practice (staffing, assessment, reviews, etc.) is surprisingly similar.

CMHTs are not the only model for provision of local services. In the US President Kennedy's 1963 'Community Mental Health Centers Construction Act' established community mental health centres. These were ambitious, relatively large units aiming to reduce fragmentation of care and provide a range of services including day care, assessment, treatment, outreach, and preventative and educational services for mental health. They were over-ambitious and proved impossible to staff and run and soon contracted to focus on day care and clinics. The model has functioned well in the Netherlands and in some parts of Europe.

Day hospitals

Day hospitals (in tandem with general hospital units) were proposed as the alternative to mental hospital care but have been overtaken somewhat by events. The need for them never fully materialized as CMHTs developed. Many of the anxiety and depression treatments they were planned for were delivered by CMHT staff with their newly acquired skills. Effective outreach to support more severely ill patients has also reduced the need for them. Day centres on the other hand (providing social, rather than health care) continue to flourish. They reduce the isolation and loneliness experienced by so many mentally ill people, particularly in large anonymous cities.

Stigma and social integration

The first twenty years of the move to community care are generally considered something of a global success. Patients who did not need to be in expensive, gloomy mental hospitals got out of them and found more rewarding lives. The support offered them by CMHTs was effective but light-touch. As mental hospitals began to close, however, patients with increasingly severe disabilities were discharged. Closures often ran far ahead of the provision of adequate alternative services, in particular, affordable local housing. Many patients became homeless (particularly in the US where this became a national scandal). Living in squalor on the streets they became a reproach to us all and often victims of petty crime and exploitation. The picture was, of course, very varied. Some states in the US had quickly developed sophisticated and admirable social provision and this was true of much of Europe. However, major cities (London, Rome, New York, Los Angeles) have struggled to cope and generally not succeeded

Changes in legislation motivated by concern for civil liberties, which prevent hospitalization unless there is evidence of immediate danger (as in New York and California), exacerbated this problem. Very disabled patients rejected hospital even if there was a bed for them and the new laws wouldn't permit their compulsion. It is telling that patients who have experienced both prefer living in poverty and insecurity on the street to being in a relatively comfortable hospital ward. This can't simply be written off as lack of insight – most of us value personal freedom and choice above comfort. However, the sight of 'bag-ladies' and homeless, obviously mentally unwell individuals on our streets presents a broad moral challenge for which we have no easy answer.

Stigma

Stigma has been proposed as one of the main burdens of mental illness and there are now international programmes aimed at reducing it. Stigma is manifest by our wish to avoid specific individuals ('establish social distance') and in its most extreme form to expel or banish them. The mentally ill have always been stigmatized, as have sufferers from many illnesses in the past. While the more extreme manifestations of stigma such as the leper's bell or branding people are lost in ancient history, discrimination and neglect still leave the mentally ill denied full social acceptance. Discrimination in jobs and housing is common. There is evidence that stigma against the mentally ill is less in younger people than in their elders. This is clearly an encouraging finding but its cause is unclear. Does the current younger generation understand mental illness better, having been more exposed to it? Or do people simply become more intolerant with age? Hopefully the former.

We usually try to avoid (i.e. 'stigmatize') people who we think pose a risk to us. In the past the fear was mainly of infection (leprosy, tuberculosis, etc.) but with mental illness it is of frightening or dangerous behaviour. It would be misleading to deny that mental illness is associated with a raised risk of violence. For most patients that risk is to themselves (suicide and self-harm) but individuals with psychosis are still about four times more likely to threaten or hurt others than non mentally ill individuals. This seems a lot but it represents a tiny risk as only 2–3 per cent of the population suffers from such disorders. The real risk to most of us is from otherwise healthy but intoxicated young men. Yet most countries are preoccupied with this risk, usually driven by high-profile cases of homicide by the mentally ill. In some cases this has led to new legislation, often taking its name from the victim (e.g. Kendra's law in the US). In the UK wholesale reform of the mental health services has been ignited by two infamous homicides, one by a neglected individual with schizophrenia and one by a chaotic drug abusing man with a severe personality disorder. Similar reforms have been initiated in Sweden after the murder of their Foreign Minister Anna Lindh.

While each of these individual incidents is a tragedy for all involved, they really do not amount to an epidemic. In England, for example, homicide by the mentally ill has remained constant at about 160 a year for the last 40 years (while homicide by the non mentally ill has increased from just over 300 a year in 1980 to over 800 in 2000). Most of these 'mental illness' homicides occur within the family or are by individuals with personality disorders often complicated by drug and alcohol misuse (not what most of us typically think of as 'mental illness'). However the fear of random assault by a psychotic individual, 'prematurely discharged from a mental hospital', exerts a remarkably powerful hold on public opinion. In the UK you are more likely to be killed by a speeding police car than by a mentally ill stranger.

Social consensus and the post-modern society

Concern with risk and its avoidance have been suggested as core features of a post-modern society. As common core values recede, protecting our individual survival and well-being becomes a dominant preoccupation. Whether or not one finds this argument convincing it is undeniable that Western societies are increasingly individualistic with less social consensus and greater risk-consciousness. The emphasis of the 1940s and 1950s on shared social capital such as public schooling and health care has given way in varying degrees to a consumerist approach with an emphasis on personalized care. This has reflected, and in turn been driven by, massively increased social mobility both locally and internationally. Families have also become less central to how we function as adults and less stable in themselves.

Modern industrial societies are rarely 'homogeneous' – there are large sections of society with quite differing origins, religions, values, and ethnicity. Despite its obvious benefits this can make psychiatry very difficult. Differing lifestyles and behaviour are accepted as choices and tolerated as long as they do not infringe the next person's liberties. Most of us value these freedoms very highly. An increasing tolerance of varied lifestyle choices however can mean a reduced sensitivity to mental illness. When you can choose to dress and behave almost any way you want, it is harder to realize when somebody's strange dress and behaviour are not simply self-expression but part of an illness. The over-active, disinhibited behaviour of manic patients is regularly misinterpreted as simply irresponsible or exhibitionist.

Increasing uncertainty about social norms has been complicated by a vast increase in alcohol and recreational drug consumption in Western societies. Intoxication usually makes mental illnesses worse and their treatment more difficult. It also significantly complicates the recognition of mental illness – it is tragically common to assess a young student who has been unwell for months but whose room-mates attributed it all to drug use and so delayed getting help.

Stigma, an exaggerated sense of risk from the mentally ill, family break-up, high social mobility, and increasing levels of drug and alcohol use all combine to make community care of the mentally ill much more difficult than it was when the process started. This is reflected in a small but widespread rise in compulsory treatment and a modest increase in 'reinstitutionalization'. This is balanced by a much more sophisticated and embedded respect for individual rights than would have been conceivable a generation ago. We are likely to experience continued soul-searching about community care and probably some rebalancing of the institution/community emphasis. A large-scale return to long-stay institutions is fairly unlikely in the coming years. Community care in one form or another is with us for the foreseeable future.

Chapter 4
Psychoanalysis and psychotherapy

Psychotherapy means different things to different people. Literally it means 'treatment of the mind', though it can be read as 'treatment *by* the mind'. I will use this second understanding (otherwise all psychiatric activity would be psychotherapy and we would be no further forward). In this chapter psychotherapy will include any deliberate, structured use of the *relationship* between a therapist and patient to help that patient to change or better understand his or herself. Psychotherapy is usually conducted by talking, hence the current expression 'talking treatments', but in some therapies words are not the crucial element and in some the 'dialogue' is internal.

How is psychotherapy different from normal kindness?

Much of what characterizes psychotherapy characterizes normal life. We all try to help our friends and family by being supportive and talking things through when they are upset. Many asylum doctors spent time in supportive conversations with their patients aiming to calm them and restore reason. This was broadly psychotherapeutic in aim. What is special about psychotherapies, however, is that there is an explicit *agreement*, almost a contract, between patient and therapist to set time aside to *concentrate* on it. They also follow a known and agreed approach, with clarity about what will happen and how long it will take.

The National Health Service in England calls psychotherapy 'talking treatments' or 'psychological treatments' to avoid old sectarian arguments about what is 'true' psychotherapy. It has a rather helpful hierarchy:

Type A comprises simple psychotherapeutic understanding employed during any treatment (e.g. counselling and support from a doctor prescribing antidepressants).

Type B involves dedicated sessions devoted exclusively to psychological understanding and emotional support. These use general psychotherapeutic principles but don't follow a strict theory or have a prescribed number of sessions. An example would be a nurse having regular meetings with a depressed patient on the ward to talk through her situation.

Type C treatments are 'psychotherapy proper'. Here the therapist has a recognized psychotherapy training and there is a clear, shared undertaking to pursue a specified course of that psychotherapy.

I've laboured this because some of the older psychotherapies are more evident in Type A and Type B treatments and are overlooked when not used as 'proper' Type C psychotherapies.

Sigmund Freud and the origins of psychoanalysis

No story of psychotherapy can ignore Sigmund Freud. Love him or loathe him, he is a towering figure who has radically altered not just psychotherapy but how much of the Western world thinks. We met him in Chapter 2, forced to leave his research and make a living for himself in private practice in Vienna. Most of his clientele was 'neurotic' and most was female. The commonest problems he saw were either 'neurasthaenia' (lack of motivation, mild depression) or a series of ostensibly physical complaints (paralyses, pains, seizures, etc.) for which there was no identifiable physical cause. Before reaching Freud they would have been subject to exhaustive medical examinations and treatments without benefit.

In over 50 years and 24 volumes of writing, Freud's ideas changed significantly and they are sometimes contradictory. The outline that follows is, of necessity, simplified and partial but there are many detailed and accessible introductions (e.g. Anthony Storr's *Freud: A Very Short Introduction*).

Freud's thinking was heavily influenced by the scientific models that surrounded him. Darwin's *Origin of Species* had located mankind squarely in the natural world (not a special divine creation) so the mind became a legitimate subject for scientific investigation. The laws of thermodynamics (which gave rise to much of 20th-century physics) dominated scientific thinking then. These proposed that energy is never lost – simply transformed. Nineteenth-century Europe was economically booming; its industry driven by mechanical innovations such as trains, factory presses, ships' engines, all based on harnessing 'conserved energy'. Whether water, steam, or internal combustion engines, they all demonstrated the enormous power of damming up energy and channelling its escape through a restricted outlet. Freud's ideas of the human mind are shot through with this metaphor – whether blocked instinctual drives or repressed memories, he believed our greatest destructive and creative achievements stemmed from forces denied their natural release.

The unconscious and free association

If the laws of energy conservation applied to the mind then new ideas and feeling had to come from somewhere. Freud observed the impact of releasing 'unconscious' forces after visiting the French neurologist Charcot who used hypnosis to cure hysterical disorders such as fits or mutism. Freud initially found hypnosis and suggestion successful with many of his patients but the results were only temporary. He encouraged them, under hypnosis, to recall the events leading up to their illness and concluded that traumatic memories were the cause of many of their maladies.

His conclusion from this was that patients are unaware of much of their 'thinking' – that some mental processes were *unconscious*. The harder one tried to remember the harder it got. Freud responded with the technique of 'free association' – encouraging the patient to stop trying to remember and instead say whatever came into their mind. Through these 'random' remarks, supplemented by recounting dreams, repressed thoughts leaked out in obscure ways (you can almost see him imagining steam driving pistons). The analyst used his own unconscious to 'listen' to these remarks, detecting patterns and so directing the patient to the source of their troubles. Hence a 'Freudian slip' is when someone reveals their true thoughts by mistake. Freud became obsessed with the need not to interfere with this free association. The 'blank screen' therapist should reveal nothing about themselves, often sitting behind the patient and never answering questions or giving reassurance. It is hard to imagine, looking at the picture of his consulting room, and knowing about the controversy that accompanied him throughout his life, how Freud could ever believe he was a blank screen.

Nineteenth-century bourgeois Vienna was a very inhibited society. Not surprisingly many of the unconscious conflicts that Freud uncovered were sexual. Initially he believed that his patients had been sexually abused but he changed to a belief that these descriptions were more often fantasies and wish-fulfilments. He went on to propound his theory of infantile sexuality – that even very small children have strong 'sexual' feelings about their parents. This, of course, caused uproar, and in many circles still does. The language is clumsy but the ideas do help make some sense of the intense and powerful dynamics children set up in families. The Oedipus Complex is his most famous construct. Freud proposed

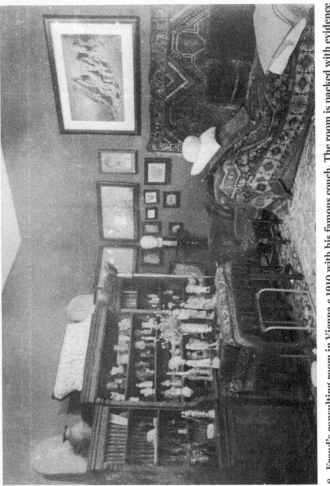

8. Freud's consulting room in Vienna c.1910 with his famous couch. The room is packed with evidence of Freud's preoccupation with ancient Egypt and mythology

that at about 3 years old the young boy desires his mother and sees his father as a rival for her affections (based on the Greek myth of Oedipus who killed his father and married his mother). Put like that it is pretty unhelpful, but it is an insightful way to understand how some people never learn to share important relationships. In the process of striving for exclusive intimacy they destroy what they want most. It made sense of many of the patients Freud saw (as it does even today).

Ego, id, and superego

Freud originally believed that the conscious mind was entirely rational and contrasted with the more primitive, less logical, unconscious mental processes. This may explain some of the exaggerated terminology he used when discussing it. However he was struck by the brutal, punitive consciences of some of his patients. How could something as noble as conscience drive a patient to suicide through guilt? His solution was to describe the conscience as derived from both conscious thoughts and also from powerful unconscious remnants of parental and social demands. His map of the mind expanded from two areas (unconscious and conscious) to three. He called the primitive unconscious the id ('it'), the conscious mind the ego ('I') and the conscience the superego (literally 'over I'). All of these terms are now in common use.

Defence mechanisms

Early psychoanalysis was about enabling the patient to discover repressed conflicts. Initially Freud and his growing band of colleagues thought that this was sufficient. However, as analyses got longer and more complex, analysts encountered 'resistance' where patients appeared to block change using various psychological defence mechanisms. One of the most troublesome 'resistances' for Freud was that patients kept falling in love with him (or at the least seeing him as a father figure). At one level this helps – if the patient likes you they are more likely to do what you ask. However, these strong feelings (he called them 'transference' because he thought they were *transferred* from important figures in the patient's past life) made the exploration of free association almost impossible. Having initially seen transference as exclusively a problem Freud began to exploit it in the analysis. This 'analysis of defence mechanisms' became an essential part of the treatment.

There were certainly many blind alleys in Freud's work – no surprise in a man who wrote so much. He made us aware of the power of unacknowledged thoughts and how the past can continue to haunt lives. Perhaps more importantly he showed that a brave attempt to confront and understand the origins of the misery (not simply to offer support and comfort) can lead to real liberation and relief. He also (against his own wishes, no doubt) showed how an honestly entered reflective human relationship can itself be the tool for recovery from quite severe mental illnesses.

Freud was a pessimist (particularly after the carnage of the First World War) and never promised happiness. The aim of psychoanalysis, he wrote, was to help a patient 'to work and to love'. No more, no less. The rigidity and grandiosity of many of his successors has tarnished his reputation. His claims to have been a scientist are questionable and his treatment, psychoanalysis, is under siege for its failure to prove effectiveness. However, he has probably contributed as much to understanding and tolerance in the care of the mentally ill as any other individual. His insistence on taking the patient's past seriously and his vivid metaphors for mental processes appeal to therapists and patients alike. They have formed the basis for a humane working relationship for which he deserves more credit than is currently his lot.

Jung

Freud collected about him a glittering band of followers. As often with such creative groups there were tensions, conflicts, and schisms. Several took the approach in differing directions and their individual fames have waxed and waned. Probably *Carl-Gustav Jung* (1875–1961) has had the most lasting influence. While Freud called himself a 'Godless Jew' with little sense of the spiritual or transcendent, Jung's theories were more mystical. They included such constructions as a racial unconscious with 'archetypes' (symbolic figures which we all share). Jung also emphasized the importance of opposites in the human personality and how a 'shadow self' develops from aspects of our personality that we fail to acknowledge. Jung probably suffered a psychotic breakdown himself and drew on some of these deeply irrational experiences. Unlike Freud he believed that therapy could promote deep personal fulfilment and his approach is attractive to those who work with very ill patients and in artistic circles. Jung's most persisting contribution, however, is probably his elaboration of the *introvert* and *extrovert* personality types. These have entered common language and are in daily usage by millions unfamiliar with even his name.

Psychodynamic psychotherapy

Psychoanalysis was closely associated with Jewish practitioners in its infancy and became a target for Nazi persecution in the 1930s. As a result most practitioners had to leave and most moved to the US, England, and South America. In all of these places their work and teaching came to have an enormous influence on psychiatry – much more than in their native German-speaking countries.

The Second World War put extra demands on psychoanalysts who turned their attention to traumatized soldiers and, surprisingly, the understanding of organizations (in particular the army). Out of this arose group analysis and group therapies where patients were treated in small groups of 5–8 so that they benefited from solidarity and support as well as insight. Group work led to the development of the therapeutic community (see Chapter 3) where analytical and psychological insights are applied to running a unit (rather than individual treatments). This informal, communal approach (with staff and patients sharing many of the tasks of running the place) was called 'sociotherapy' and has become a standard feature of modern psychiatric practice, drug rehabilitation units, and some prisons.

The endlessness of classic psychoanalysis (often taking several years at three to five sessions a week) has been strongly criticized. It is prohibitively expensive and many believed that shorter therapies would focus the mind better and improve outcomes. Typical 'short-term' therapies now last three to six months with weekly sessions of an hour. Interpersonal therapy focuses on relationships and cognitive analytical therapy uses specific exercises like letter writing and prescription of homework as part of the treatment. While still maintaining strict professional boundaries therapists are increasingly more active.

These are usually called 'psychodynamic' psychotherapies because they attribute such importance to dynamic interactions between the past and the present and between conscious and unconscious processes. The individual's life story, their 'narrative', is central to understanding and resolving their problems. All require the therapist to hold back from giving too much direct advice so that the patient can, with guidance, find their own solutions. These therapies are routinely combined with other psychiatric treatments (antidepressants, hospital care, etc.).

Non-specific factors in psychotherapy

Most psychodynamic psychotherapists are intensely loyal to their model, convinced of the specificity of their treatment. Unfortunately the evidence is against them. There is depressingly little research into psychodynamic psychotherapies (unlike cognitive behavioural therapies) but what there is makes interesting reading. Experienced therapists who follow their training closely do much better than novices, or those who apply their model loosely. However, *which* model doesn't seem to matter so much – they are all about equally effective. Most of this research confirms the crucial importance of establishing a good therapeutic relationship.

The qualities of a good therapist transcend the different schools of thought. The essential ingredients are *accurate empathy* (the therapist must really understand what the patient is going through, it is not enough just to feel sorry for them), *unconditional regard* (the therapist has to like and respect the patient, you can't do therapy with someone you really dislike), and *non-possessive warmth* (the therapist must be able to show warmth without making the patient feel beholden to them). These insights are particularly useful in psychiatric practice. Matching patients and therapists really does matter – not all of us can get on with everyone. To work with violent or sexual offenders, for instance, requires a particularly tolerant and forgiving individual.

Existential and experimental psychotherapies

Several schools of psychotherapy have evolved which utilize the techniques of psychodynamic psychotherapy without accepting the theory. Existential psychotherapy, as its name suggests, makes no assumptions about what people 'should be like' but focuses on helping the patient express their identity in their own chosen way. Existential psychotherapies have some affinity with Jungian approaches and have become more popular as society becomes less rigid and conformist.

Freud's patients usually knew what their families and society expected of them and were anguished because they could not achieve it. In the early 21st century we are more likely to experience aimlessness and emptiness rather than guilt at not living up to expectations. Alienation and confusion are now the dominant complaints so psychotherapies have become more structured to provide boundaries and containment.

These more here-and-now therapies blend imperceptibly into the personal growth movement. It can be difficult sometimes to decide whether a gestalt therapy or encounter group is a *treatment* to reduce suffering or an *exercise* to increase personal happiness and fulfilment. Perhaps it doesn't matter what the purpose is so much as who gets it. There can be little doubt that depressed and demoralized psychiatric patients benefit greatly from activities such as these which improve general morale and self-esteem. In the treatments of self-harming young women, addressing self-esteem directly may be one of the most effective interventions.

Psychodynamic psychotherapies are currently under attack in psychiatry. They are criticized for inadequate research to establish that they really do work. Also, the requirement for therapists to undergo treatment themselves and to continue with supervision throughout their professional lives compromises objectivity and smacks of a 'cult' rather than a profession. Some research has been conducted in the short-term dynamic therapies and their results are generally good. However, more detailed studies to identify which aspects are effective, and which redundant, remain to be done. The opportunity may even have passed. So many of the core features of psychodynamic psychotherapy are now absorbed into routine care (the Type A and B treatments referred to above) that their contribution as specific treatments may be difficult to isolate and evaluate.

The strength of criticism is not surprising as psychoanalysis really did oversell itself. In America (North and South) between 1940 and 1970 it virtually drove all other thinking out of mental health care – most people thought that a psychiatrist *was* a psychoanalyst. Psychotic patients, for whom analysis had little to offer, were neglected, as were the basic skills of diagnosis and treatment. Critics accused American psychiatry in this period, with its high status and expanding workforce, of simply turning its back on the severely mentally ill and on science altogether. President Kennedy tried to refocus the profession in the early 1960s but without success and it required the pharmacological revolution to achieve it.

A more scientific and self-critical psychiatry, obliged to establish itself with hard won research data, has taken its revenge on psychoanalysis (and some would say is now making many of the same mistakes – Chapter 6).

The newer psychotherapies and counselling

The last 40 years have seen the development of a whole series of new psychotherapies that are radically different. They pay far less attention to understanding the past. The therapists are usually more directive – they give instructions and opinions, not just further encouragement to the patient to continue reflecting. Many involve specific exercises and 'homework' that is reviewed in sessions. They last months not years. The psychotherapist acts much like any other mental health professional and avoids the mystique surrounding psychodynamic therapists.

Person-centred (often called Rogerian) counselling is one such approach. The distinction between counselling and psychotherapy is variable and unclear. Counselling is often offered at times of personal crisis to people we would not usually consider as 'ill'. Its aims are more modest than those of formal therapies. It draws on the characteristics of a good therapist outlined above, and provides a 'safe space' for the individual to explore their concerns. Here the therapist *is* non-directive. They rarely give opinions or advise the patient what to do or think, and often simply repeat the patient's last phrase as encouragement to continue reflecting. Counselling is a skill highly prized by many mental health professionals and clearly valued by patients.

Family and systems therapies and crisis intervention

Family therapies have become very important in the treatment of psychiatrically ill children. Family therapists generally avoid implying a role for the family in causing the illness (see Chapter 5), but sometimes it is impossible for a patient to get better unless the family changes its way of responding. In anorexia nervosa, for instance, a family may have become so anxious about their daughter's illness that they cannot allow her the freedom to take necessary risks and so mature. They may need help to back off and contain their anxiety. Sometimes the same can occur with adult patients where family therapy often helps couples shift the balance in their relationship. Family therapy usually relies on a 'systems' approach where the whole family is the focus, not the individual members.

'Behavioural family management' using a problem-solving approach helps families of schizophrenia patients. Patients break down more often if they live in highly emotional families – especially where there is tension and criticism. It may be very difficult for the family to avoid this, so the treatment is aimed at identifying flash-points in the relationships and finding alternative solutions (e.g. going into another room rather than arguing back). This has been shown to reduce breakdown rates by almost as much as medicine, but is protracted and difficult to do.

Crisis therapy is in here with systems therapies because it deals with immediate issues. You don't have to dig around in crisis or family therapy – it's all there in front of you. Crisis therapy is dramatic, often ultra short-term, and handles strong emotions, often with limited attention to their origins. While the family therapies are generally well established there remain doubts about crisis therapy. Some researchers suggest, for example, that debriefing after trauma can even make things worse. Presumably it interferes with the healthy processes of forgetting distressing events.

Behaviour therapy

Behaviour therapy principles are about as different from psychodynamic psychotherapy as it is possible to be. They are based on learning theory which made a virtue of removing 'consciousness' from the equation – change is explained by reflex learning. Behaviour therapy is indelibly associated with B. F. Skinner who demonstrated that you could train rats in quite complex behaviours simply by rewarding the behaviour you wanted ('operant conditioning') or, alternatively, 'punishing' the behaviour you wanted to stop. Behaviour is 'shaped' in small steps, one at a time. The unique aspect of behaviour therapy is that it is irrelevant whether the subject agrees or even knows what is going on – the learning is completely unconscious.

Behaviour therapy can be staggeringly effective – think how easy it is to ride a bike and yet you probably have never 'consciously' learnt. You just tried it and each time it started to go wrong your body compensated, and now you are supremely skilled. Behaviour therapy works like that. It has proved particularly effective in treatments for individuals with learning disabilities and with children. A simple example of operant conditioning is the bell-and-pad system for nocturnal enuresis (bed wetting). A bell rings as soon as the pad gets wet, waking the patient. Over time he starts to wake up when his (it is usually his) bladder is full, as that sensation becomes associated with the bell and being woken. This successful treatment is widely used despite contradictory beliefs that bed wetting is either evidence of neurotic problems or, the opposite, that it is predominantly genetic.

Behaviour therapy is extensively used for phobias and for obsessive compulsive disorders. The patient is gradually exposed to the feared stimulus (e.g. a dirty hand for someone with obsessions about germs) while restricting avoidance and monitoring anxiety to ensure it remains tolerable. In practice behaviour therapists still take detailed histories because, without a good therapeutic relationship, patients drop out of treatment.

Cognitive behavioural therapy

Cognitive behavioural therapy could be considered a sophisticated extension of behaviour therapy, although it could also be viewed as an adaptation of psychodynamic psychotherapy. It lies somewhere between the two. It was developed by an American psychiatrist,

Aaron Beck. He was a psychoanalytically trained psychiatrist who found a proportion of patients did not benefit from his psychoanalysis. On the whole they were people who valued mastery of their symptoms more than understanding them. His exploration, particularly of depression, convinced him that it was unconscious and pathological *thoughts* as much as feelings that were trapping his patients. He developed a therapy to enable patients to identify 'automatic negative thoughts' (self-critical, self-defeating beliefs and conclusions) and to train them in how to challenge and contradict them.

His method emphasized 'Socratic Dialogue'. Socrates believed that all you needed to teach truth was to keep asking the right questions and people found the answers within. Whenever the patient expresses a pathological doubt – e.g. 'I got it wrong at work today. There's no future for me', the therapist asks them to explain it – 'Explain to me why there is no hope.' He contrasts the thoughts with the reality of the situation – 'Explain how it is that you're still being promoted at work then, despite these mistakes?' CBT is now an essential part of psychiatric practice and training and is a standard ingredient in the treatments of depression and anxiety. It is also being increasingly used in a whole range of disorders including schizophrenia with intractable hallucinations or delusions and also physical disorders with a significant psychological component.

Self-help

It may not be psychiatry, but the self-help movement has grown out of the psychotherapy tradition. Alcoholics Anonymous, Weight Watchers, The Depression Alliance, have all begun to apply what they have learnt, and more. Accurate empathy and unconditional regard – who better than someone who has been through it? Who less likely to condemn than someone with the same problems? Non-possessive warmth – what better source than shared suffering and real fellow-feeling? Self-help groups constitute a folk movement of our times which relieves distress and isolation and reduces stigma. Self-help books and computer programmes are increasingly available for common disorders like anxiety and depression. It is too early to judge their impact but they certainly get the popular vote.

After 200 years of psychiatry it seems strange for psychotherapy to be restricted to its own short chapter. Can it really be considered independent from psychiatry or psychiatry independent from it? Psychotherapy has been a defining characteristic of the psychiatric craft – just as a surgeon operates, a radiographer reads x-rays, an obstetrician delivers a baby. Asylum doctors of 150 years ago spent time talking with distressed patients to bring understanding, comfort, and relief. In the second half of the 20th century this personal relationship was why most staff came into the profession. Yet as we start the 21st century psychiatry and psychotherapy are increasingly considered as parallel activities. Is psychiatry changing fundamentally? Time will tell if they are to grow together again or to continue to pursue increasingly independent paths. Some of the forces driving these changes will occupy us in succeeding chapters.

Chapter 5
Psychiatry under attack – inside and out

Psychiatry has always been controversial – there never was an extended 'Golden Age' of peace and tranquillity when everyone was in agreement. You probably bought this book after some heated discussion about the rights and wrongs of something psychiatrists do. Because it deals with the mind, and because psychiatrists can act against our wishes, it will always generate a degree of suspicion and fear. And it isn't good enough simply to put this down to ignorance and say that if people knew more they wouldn't have such concerns. There are very real questions to be asked about psychiatry – both about its legitimacy, its status as 'just another medical specialty', and also about how it is practised. The power of modern medicine invariably brings ethical challenges and controversies and psychiatry has its fair share. These will be taken up more in Chapter 6. This chapter will focus on the contradictions and tensions which are *inherent* in psychiatry, that stem from its very nature, rather than problems with practice.

Mind-body dualism

The French philosopher René Descartes (1596–1650) is often blamed for how we distinguish between the mind and the body in Western thought (often referred to as 'Cartesian dualism'). His 'cogito ergo sum' ('I think therefore I am') is snappy and memorable; it expresses his scepticism about certainty in knowing about the material world. It is hard to understand why he has been singled out for all the 'blame' for an issue which exercised most of his empiricist philosopher contemporaries. He didn't *invent* the problem of the mind; he simply put some of the issues better and they remain essentially unresolved 350 years later. What the mind is, and how it interacts with the material world, still remain mysteries. Most of us *do* think there is a difference and most of us accept that there *is* an interaction. We have to live our lives believing we can directly influence the material world (e.g. I decide to stretch out my arm and expect to turn on the computer). We also need to believe that we can know the minds of others (e.g. I'm sure that you will go to the library or hand in your essay). Without these beliefs we would effectively be paralysed.

The mind–body question is unavoidable in psychiatry. The relationship between the mind and the brain is *the* big issue. It would be simple if psychiatry were just about 'brain diseases' in the way that nephrology is about kidney diseases or cardiology is about heart diseases. Psychiatry, however, is concerned with 'mental' illnesses. We know that many mental illnesses involve disorders of the brain (e.g. disturbances in transmitter chemicals between cells in depression and schizophrenia) but not all brain diseases are mental illnesses or the responsibility of psychiatrists. Multiple sclerosis and Parkinson's disease are both undeniably brain diseases but it is neurologists, not psychiatrists, who deal with them. These neurological disorders often *cause* psychiatric problems, just as a wide range of physical disorders can. Many psychiatric disorders include physical symptoms (e.g. tiredness and pain), just as physical disorders include psychiatric symptoms (e.g. depression, anxiety, and even hallucinations).

Psychiatric disorders are those where the main disturbances are in thoughts, feelings, and behaviour (Chapter 1). Physical diseases don't just have physical causes and cures and mental diseases have mental causes and cures. Illnesses can have physical causes and even physical cures (e.g. a depression caused entirely by Parkinson's disease which is effectively treated by antidepressant tablets) and still be 'mental illnesses'. The division is based on the *main* disturbance and on the *skills* needed to help the patient. 'Mental disorders are brain disorders' has been a popular slogan with some psychiatrists and patient groups. Its purpose is to emphasize the similarity between mental and physical illnesses, reducing stigma and blame. These are admirable goals but it is an over-simplification. Psychiatry has to struggle with an ambiguity fought out on two main battlegrounds.

Nature versus nurture: do families cause mental illness?

Whether you're tall or short, whether you're good at sport or hopeless, most of us believe this depends on a mixture of our genes (the biological potential we were born with) and our upbringing (our diet, exercise regime, even the sort of school we went to). Nothing controversial in that. The moment we mention psychology, however, the balloon goes up. Is IQ inherited or could everyone do just as well with the same opportunities? Is personality or criminality something we're born with or can we change it? Can we avoid depression by healthy living? Few issues polarize us as much as how changeable we believe human behaviour to be. The disagreements are not just calm, academic ones but fuel (and are fuelled by) political and social beliefs reflecting fundamentally different worldviews.

Psychiatry originally was very much at home in the 'nature' camp – mental illnesses ran in families and were inherited weaknesses. It was our job to ameliorate them and make life as bearable as possible, hoping for a speedy recovery. Freud and his followers began to change all that, shifting the balance to 'nurture'. Psychoanalysis is firmly based on the belief that what happens to us in early life, and the memory of those experiences, is the *cause* of many illnesses. Even more convincing, Freud showed that addressing those memories could *cure* some mental illnesses. So an individual's personal history (their 'narrative') wasn't just the context for understanding their illness but possibly its origin.

Psychoanalysis dominated psychiatric thinking and training from the 1940s to the 1970s. The attraction of psychoanalysis to the Americas should come as no shock. After all, these societies were established by those who escaped the pessimistic fatalism of Europe with its fixed social orders and hereditary monarchies and aristocracies. Those who moved west were those who rejected this and grasped the opportunity for each individual to shape their own future. No surprise then that they espoused a psychology that enshrined this capacity for growth, where the individual could overcome early limitations and forge their own destiny. The role of nurture and experience was strengthened by observations of battle trauma in both world wars (Chapter 3). The revelation of the eugenic and racist policies of Nazi Germany (including the liquidation of 'genetically inferior' psychiatric patients) finally guaranteed nurture's moral unassailability.

An attraction of emphasizing nurture is that it holds out much greater possibility of cure. If mental illnesses are essentially *caused* by relationships then they should be curable by relationships (i.e. psychotherapy). However, the downside of this approach is its potential for blame – in particular blaming parents. Freud himself quickly realized these risks when he began to suspect that the reported sexual abuse by parents (which he originally considered the cause of his patients' neuroses) might be fantasies. The great German psychopathologist and philosopher Jaspers pointed out that, while understanding the personal relevance of symptoms was essential in psychiatry, it was not the same as understanding what *caused* the illness. Such fine distinctions have not, however, generally characterized this debate publically.

The origins of schizophrenia

This controversy has raged most fiercely over the origins of schizophrenia. Schizophrenia had always been known to run in families and it had been observed that these families could seem 'odd' (eccentric or withdrawn), often with strained or intensely over-involved relationships. As schizophrenia is a disorder expressed in thinking and relating there is an obvious possible link between it and early upbringing. Family life is, after all, conducted through thinking and relating and aims to equip the growing child with skills in these areas. As psychoanalytical thinking was applied to schizophrenia (something that Freud explicitly avoided) a number of theories were proposed, some of which had enormous influence and have entered the language.

The 'schizophrenogenic mother'

The most notorious (and probably the most damaging) of these was that of the cold, hostile, and yet controlling parent – the 'schizophrenogenic mother' (literally 'schizophrenia-causing mother'). This was proposed by the analyst Frieda Fromm-Reichmann who, along with Harry Stack Sullivan, engaged in long-term intensive psychoanalysis with hospitalized schizophrenia patients in the USA. Her most famous patient, Joanna Greenberg, later described her experiences in her best-selling autobiographical novel *I Never Promised You a Rose-Garden*.

Fromm-Reichmann described a powerful, but cold and rejecting mother figure who bound the patient close to her, preventing the growth of healthy independence and sense of self. Schizophrenia was then understood as a disorder of 'ego-development' resulting in weak personal boundaries (hence the confusion of internal and external experiences in hallucinations). Fromm-Reichmann's conclusions are preposterous by current standards. She based them entirely on her patients' reports in analysis and never actually bothered to meet or interview the mothers. It is reputed that her ideas derived from the analysis of only 11 patients. Despite its early rejection within the profession, the conviction lives on that families can 'cause' schizophrenia. This has led to endless self-blame by parents and, in some circumstances, their rejection and exclusion by mental health staff.

The 'double-bind'

The anthropologist Gregory Bateson proposed that persistent, logically faulty, and contradictory communication with a child prevented it forming a proper sense of itself and its relationships to the external world. Bateson was influenced by Bertrand Russell and A. N. Whitehead's mathematical writings. One of their proposals was that the number which designated a series of numbers could not itself be a member of that series – as the designating number was of a 'logically different order'. Bateson said that there were similarly logically different levels of communication and that we sent messages to each other (often in an oblique manner) where one part of the message indicated how the main part should be understood. He called these oblique messages 'meta-communications' (i.e. communications about communication). Typically meta-communications were emotional and non-verbal and became family assumptions (e.g. 'mother can only love her children and always feel positive about them').

Bateson called it a double-bind when the non-verbal message and verbal message contradicted each other (e.g. an obviously angry mother saying she didn't mind at all that the child had broken a glass and holding her arms out for an embrace). A double-bind required three components: a clear simple message, a contradictory meta-communication, and an absolute ban on the contradiction being acknowledged. All three were necessary but it was probably the family culture of denying the contradiction that was most pathological. After all, all families give contradictory and confusing messages. The term 'double-bind' is now used loosely to imply any contradictory communication but Bateson's theory was much more precise.

These theories have all been conclusively demolished by careful scientific examination. One approach was to get independent researchers to listen to tapes of families with and without schizophrenia and rate the occurrence of double-binds, or to interview families and rate them for coldness, hostility, over-involvement, etc. Reliable differences were simply not found. Adoption studies, however, delivered the coup de grace. Very rigorous studies of children adopted away at birth to healthy families found rates of schizophrenia when they grew up just as high as if they had been brought up with their schizophrenic mother. Similarly twins adopted away at birth to different families demonstrated the same difference in rates between identical and non-identical twins found in those brought up in their natural families. None of these risks are 100 per cent and clearly upbringing and environment have quite a lot of influence.

While family influence as the *cause* of schizophrenia has been conclusively dismissed it remains implicated in the *course* of the illness. Individuals with schizophrenia in highly emotionally charged families are likely to break down more often. This could, of course, be because families with more severely ill members are more stressful (see Chapter 4). However, training families to respond less emotionally does reduce the rate of breakdown, so high expressed emotion probably does have an effect.

Social and peer-group pressure

While family influence has been questioned, wider social influences have received increasing recognition in the last half century. For example, the rise in eating disorders (anorexia nervosa and bulimia) has spread from the West, closely tracking the cultural ideal of thinness in women. The epidemic of self-harm (particularly overdosing and cutting in younger women) is clearly affected by group norms and expectations. Local outbreaks can often be linked to specific events such as suicide attempts in TV soap operas.

Alcohol and drug use are highly variable between different cultural groups (both between and within nations) and the power of group expectations on such behaviours is undeniable. These are enormously important public health issues and the status of these behaviours as 'mental illnesses' will be picked up again in Chapter 6.

Evolutionary psychology

The fading relevance of the nature–nurture argument has recently been revived by the rise of evolutionary psychology. A more sophisticated understanding of Darwinian evolution (survival of the fittest) has led to theories about the possible evolutionary value of some psychiatric disorders. A simplistic view would predict that all mental illnesses with a genetic component should lower survival and ought to die out. 'Inclusive fitness', however, assesses the evolutionary value of a characteristic not simply on whether it helps that *individual* to survive but whether it makes it more likely that their *offspring* will survive. Richard Dawkins's 1976 book *The Selfish Gene* gives convincing explanations of the evolutionary advantages of group support and altruism when individuals sacrifice themselves for others.

A range of speculative hypotheses have since been proposed for the evolutionary advantage of various behaviour differences and mental illnesses. Many of these draw on ethological games-theory (i.e. the benefits of any behaviour can only be understood in the context of the behaviour of other members of the group). So depression might be seen as a safe response to 'defeat' in a hierarchical group because it makes the individual withdraw from conflict while they recover. Mania, conversely, with its expansiveness and increased sexual activity, is proposed as a response to success in a hierarchical tussle promoting the propagation of that individual's genes. Changes in behaviour that look like depression and hypomania can be clearly seen in primates as they move up and down the pecking order that dominates their lives.

The habitual isolation and limited need for social contact of individuals with schizophrenia has been rather imaginatively proposed as adaptive to remote habitats with low food supplies (and also a protection against the risk of infectious diseases and epidemics). Evolutionary psychology will undoubtedly increasingly influence psychiatric thinking – many of our disorders fit poorly into a classical 'medical model'. Already it has helped establish a less either–or approach to the discussion. It is, however, a highly controversial area – not so much around mental disorders but in relation to social behaviour and particularly to gender specific behaviour. Here it is often interpreted as excusing a very male-orientated, exploitative worldview. Luckily that is someone else's battle.

Why do families blame themselves?

If so many of the family theories have been discredited why spend so much time on the issue here? Family theories in mental illness continue to exercise a remarkably powerful hold over us despite the evidence. And not just in schizophrenia but in depression, anorexia nervosa, personality disorder, drug and alcohol abuse, etc. Parents seem to have an endless capacity to blame themselves for what happens to their children (and perhaps children to blame their parents). This is probably because we need to believe it. Just as we need to believe in free will and our influence on the outside world, family members need to believe that they influence each other. If we didn't why would we bother? The evolutionary psychologists would say that parents need to believe it to invest years and years bringing up their children. We're biologically programmed to look after our children so we need some belief system to support it (just as they might say we're biologically programmed to mate and need to believe in love to support it). It is proposed that such a belief is a mechanism for sustaining our attention to our biological task.

The downside is, of course, guilt and blame. If we believe we have an influence we feel we have failed if things do not work out well. It is inescapable. Even in expressed emotion work where therapists insist emphatically that no one is to blame and that the aim is solely to find more effective coping strategies, families do feel blamed. 'If only we weren't so over-involved he would not have so many relapses.' 'Other families must have dealt with it better otherwise how would the therapist know what to advise?' For some families feeling responsible, despite the guilt, is preferable. It implies the logical consequence that there must be *something* they can do to influence the outcome. Cultures which value resignation are less likely to blame themselves (high expressed emotion is less common in India than in Europe).

The anti-psychiatry movement

Arguments over mind and brain and nature and nurture have always been part of psychiatry and are likely to remain so. They supported the most sustained and celebrated 'external' onslaught on psychiatry. This occurred during the 1960s and 1970s in what came to be called the 'anti-psychiatry movement'. The mental hospital scandals of the early 1960s and publication of Erving Goffman's *Asylums* had prepared the ground for a devastating attack. This was not to be a criticism of some of psychiatry's practices or of failures in the system; this was to be an assault on the very legitimacy of psychiatry.

The anti-psychiatry message was that psychiatry did not so much need improving as scrapping. At its best it was confused and confusing and at its worst a truly evil instrument of oppression masquerading as a benign medical practice. Three charismatic authors came to personify the movement. Two were practising psychiatrists. Their books became campus bibles in the late 1960s and the 1970s at a time of widespread student unrest and they were hugely influential in the Paris student revolt of 1968 and its international consequences.

Thomas Szasz, a Hungarian immigrant to the US, rose to fame with his book *The Myth of Mental Illness* in 1961. In this he argued that 'mental illnesses' were fabrications to deny socially deviant individuals their legal rights. He argued vigorously against involuntary treatment and for the separation of psychiatry and the state and the abolition of the insanity defence. He believed that those judged mentally ill should be treated equally and held accountable for their actions (i.e. psychotic individuals should have the right to refuse treatment and be sent to prison if they break the law, even when demonstrably unwell). He often drew on hysteria as his model of mental illness (probably reflecting his experience as a psychoanalyst in New York), which has limited the power of his case. It has been suggested that his extreme libertarian standpoint and opposition to compulsion stemmed from his experiences under Soviet occupation. He is regularly quoted by the Church of Scientology in their opposition to state run and coercive psychiatry.

Michel Foucault was a French philosopher who believed that the concept of mental illness was an aberration of the post-Enlightenment age. He objected to the classification of identities, arguing that the existence of *madness* did not entail the identity of *madman*. His book *Madness and Civilisation* challenged the very basis of psychiatric practice and cast it as repressive and controlling (rather than curing and liberating). His work had enormous influence in Continental Europe (most evident in Basaglia's reforms in Italy). However, his writing is dense and difficult to absorb and he is more often quoted than read.

The most accessible and influential of the anti-psychiatrists was R. D. Laing. A Glaswegian psychoanalyst with a brilliant mind and lucid prose style, he turned the psychiatric world upside down with a series of best-selling books. An original and impulsive man, his views changed throughout his career and like Freud he didn't feel the need to acknowledge these radical changes or explain them. His first, and most influential book, was

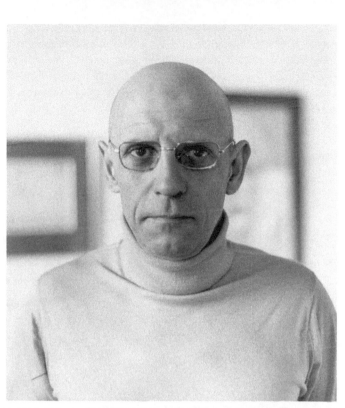

9. Michel Foucault (1926–84): French philosopher who criticized psychiatry as a repressive social force legitimizing the abuse of power

The Divided Self: An Existential Study in Sanity and Madness (1960). He called his position 'existential phenomenology' (don't ask!) and proposed that the delusional thinking of the schizophrenia patient was simply a different take on the world. He argued that this could be challenging but it was essentially creative and, with enough imagination and moral courage, could be understood. However, these different worldviews threaten our security so we seek to deny them by imposing a diagnosis and 'pathologizing' them.

The book is filled with vivid descriptions of patients Laing had treated, accompanied with the most moving and imaginative interpretations of their dilemma. The impression given of psychosis by *The Divided Self* was of a tormented and rather heroic individual communicating vivid, authentic experiences, only to be met with a cowardly and mean-spirited rejection from society. Although he did

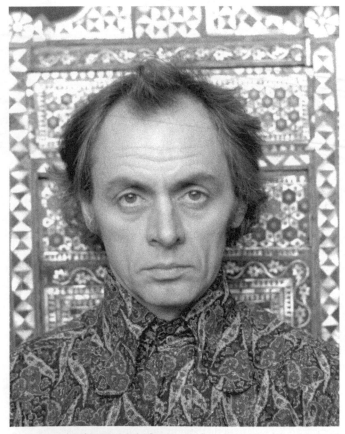

10. R. D. Laing (1927–1989): the most influential and iconic of the anti-psychiatrists of the 1960s and 1970s

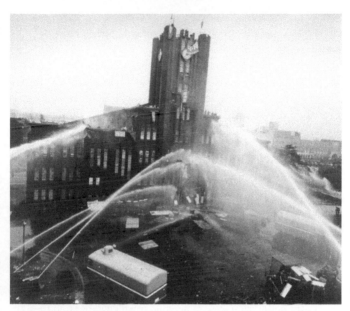

11. The remains of the administrative building, Tokyo University – students burnt it down after R. D. Laing's lecture in 1969

not deny the suffering, his was essentially a romantic view of madness which (paradoxically) increased recruitment into psychiatry at the same time that it attacked it. Like Szasz, Laing never called himself an anti-psychiatrist (a term coined by his colleague David Cooper in 1967), and continued to practise, albeit in unorthodox ways.

Laing's second 'phase' was his belief that families contributed to schizophrenia by denying the emerging identity of their child. *Sanity, Madness and the Family: Families of Schizophrenics*, with Aaron Esterson, cast schizophrenia as a response to repressive and rejecting parenting. The film inspired by it (*Family Life*, 1971) struck an international chord. Laing's third phase was inspired by his extensive experimentation with LSD, so common at that time. *The Politics of Experience and the Bird of Paradise*, published in

1967, conceived of psychosis as a psychedelic voyage of discovery in which the boundaries of perception were widened, and consciousness expanded.

Laing was an improbable candidate for such an influential role. He started his psychiatric career as an army psychiatrist. His personal life was turbulent, with several marriages and many children. As a lecturer he ranged from the inspirational to the frankly intoxicated and unintelligible. His ability to galvanize anti-establishment feeling was so powerful that after a lecture to the student body in Tokyo in 1969 they went off and set fire to the university administration building! He remained a radical until his death, aged 62, surprising all who knew him by collapsing while engaged in the outrageously bourgeois activity of playing tennis on the French Riviera.

Anti-psychiatry in the 21st century

The contradictions inherent in psychiatry which generated the anti-psychiatry movement in the 1960s and 1970s have not gone away. Mind and brain, freedom and coercion, the right to be different (perhaps even the *duty* to be different), nature and nurture remain live issues. Many (though by no means all) ex-patient groups have become militantly anti-psychiatric, often referring to themselves as 'survivors' rather than patients, clients, or service users. In Germany and Holland the state contributes to hostels and crash pads for individuals who have 'escaped' routine mental health services. The most high-profile anti-psychiatry group is probably the Church of Scientology. While much of their focus is on controversial treatments such as brain surgery and ECT (Chapter 6), they are critical of the whole endeavour. They would argue that we should avoid artificial and technological approaches to human suffering and seek alternative personal routes to relief.

Overall, however, there is now much less concerted opposition to psychiatry as a discipline. This may, in part, be due to a somewhat exaggerated faith in the rapid expansion of 'biological' explanations and an optimism that genetic and genomic advances will soon render the whole issue academic. However, while there is less conceptual opposition to psychiatry, there is no shortage of disquiet about various aspects of its practice. We turn to these now in Chapter 6.

Chapter 6
Open to abuse

Controversies in psychiatric practice

The very nature of psychiatric practice lays it open to potential misuse and abuse. It involves a highly unequal power relationship with very dependent and vulnerable patients whose opinions and complaints can so easily be dismissed as 'part of the illness'. Add to this the subjective nature of a diagnostic process which relies on psychiatrists' assessments of the patient's motives and mental state with no visible markers for diseases. The history of psychiatry doesn't inspire that much confidence either. There have been shameful episodes of political abuse, some hare-brained theories, and treatments that appear to us both dangerous and barbaric. The very visibility of modern-day psychiatry (out from behind the institutions' walls), plus a well informed public and a willingness to admit if things go wrong, is probably the greatest safeguard against such abuses. Psychiatry is also, thankfully, fully engaged in the worldwide movement of scientific, evidence-based medicine – facts and figures take precedence over authority and opinion. So while we focus in this chapter on what it can get wrong, let's not forget that it more often gets it right and that progress has been substantial.

In the public imagination the greatest risk of psychiatric abuse comes from its immense power. The evil psychiatrist is portrayed in films manipulating the minds of his victim for his own ends, taking pleasure in subjugating the distressed and suggestible. Hannibal Lecter in *Silence of the Lambs* is one such – immensely skilled at reading his victim's mind and using that power to trap and exploit them. In other films psychiatrists develop megalomaniacal delusions of using their power to rule the world.

There have been cases where this has happened on a small scale–where psychiatrists, convinced of their own infallibility, have wreaked havoc. Experiments with altering gender identity to confirm that it was socially determined is an extreme example, the mutilation of hundreds of individuals in a craze to remove sources of infection in teeth and bowels that were deemed the cause of mental illness and the wholesale use of lobotomy in the 1940s and early 1950s are others. However most of psychiatry's excesses have stemmed from the very opposite, from psychiatrists' sense of impotence and frustration turning to ever more desperate interventions to help tormented patients.

This dynamic is changing. Professions are no longer so powerful and independent. Deference and respect for authority are under global attack. The current risks in psychiatric practice may come less from professional isolation and arrogance than from social compliance. Monitoring psychiatrists may be only half of the job – we need to keep a wary eye on the other powerful players (multinational drug companies, governments, pressure groups) who can manipulate psychiatry. This is a diffuse and changing subject so what follows is just indicative.

Old sins

Like all of medicine, psychiatry's history includes what now appear dangerous and even barbaric treatments. Before being too critical think what it must have been to live at a time when early and sudden death was a constant threat and excruciating pain had to be endured, often for weeks and months on end. There were few certainties and even fewer effective treatments. What doctors were willing to do two centuries ago, and what patients were prepared to endure, have to be judged against quite different standards. Folk treatment of the mad was also far from gentle, despite our tendency to romanticize pre-industrial societies. Disabled individuals were often accepted and occasionally revered but the more disturbed were often excluded (which could mean death) or mistreated as witches or such like.

Early psychiatrists used the standard medical treatments of their time including bleeding, purging, and cupping (attaching hot cups to the back to 'draw out' toxins). The early asylums moved away from these, emphasizing moral treatments (Chapter 2), although various desperate measures were tried to calm 'furiously' agitated patients. These included cold baths (still used well into the 20th century) and a series of ingenious devices which worked by simply exhausting the patient, such as the notorious 'whirling chair'. However, the major sins of the asylum era were those of neglect – restraint rather than attention, undignified and humiliating conditions rather than active abuse.

Long-term fluctuating illnesses are particularly prone to accumulate far-fetched theories and treatments. This is a mixture of desperation and pure chance (an illness may simply recover just when some irrelevant treatment is being used). There was a vogue for removing otherwise healthy organs in the mentally ill in the late 19th century because they were thought to be the site of 'sepsis' (low grade infection). Thousands of healthy teeth and tonsils were removed and even large parts of the bowel. In Trenton State Hospital, New Jersey, Dr Henry Cotton championed this approach right up until his death in 1933 (including taking out all the teeth from his own two sons and even subjecting one to an abdominal operation). These treatments were controversial but still supported by distinguished psychiatric figures.

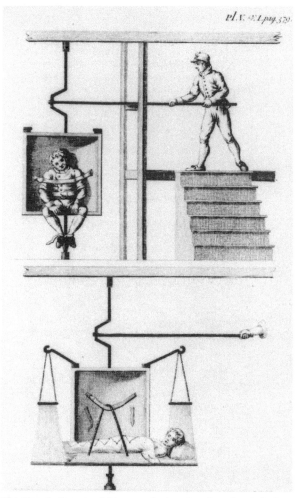

12. Whirling chair: one of the many devices developed to 'calm' over-excited patients by exhausting them

Pl. XXV.

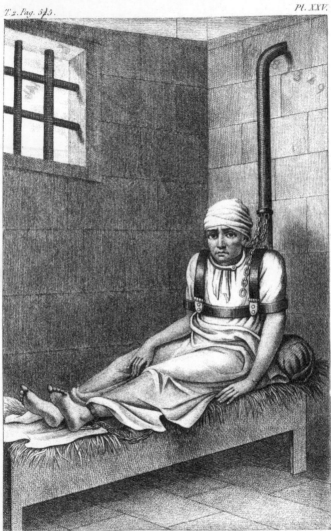

Gravé par Ambroise Tardieu.

13. **William Norris chained in Bedlam, in 1814**

The Hawthorn effect

A complicating factor is that the fuss and attention surrounding treatments can make a real difference even if the treatment itself is ineffective. This was shown with insulin coma treatment. Insulin had been long used in psychiatry to stimulate appetite and calm agitated patients (who could otherwise literally starve to death). A course of insulin comas was believed to be effective in schizophrenia and this became a common treatment from the 1930s through to the 1960s. It was a potentially dangerous treatment requiring skilled and attentive nursing – if the coma went too deep the patient could die. It was the first psychiatric treatment subject to a *controlled trial* to establish its effect. Half the patients were put into a light sleep using tranquillizers and half into an insulin coma, without the staff knowing which was which. The results were the same for both groups, forcing the conclusion that it was the nursing attention and hope inspired by the treatment that made the difference, not the insulin. The treatment was abandoned. This effect is known as the 'Hawthorn' effect and psychiatric research always has to account for enthusiasm.

Enthusiasm shouldn't be written off in psychiatry. Much of medicine may be best conducted in a dispassionate, scientific frame of mind but psychiatry requires hope and optimism from its staff. Patients have so often lost hope and need help regaining it. Hope is therapeutic in its own right as the insulin coma study indicated. Many studies have confirmed that optimism makes a difference to outcome (even in cancer patients). It can, however, lead to over-enthusiasm and treatments, including effective treatments, being given well beyond their indications.

Electro convulsive therapy and brain surgery

ECT was certainly overused after it was introduced in the 1930s right through to the 1960s. It continued to be used in schizophrenia and for disturbed behaviour although it had become clear that its main effect is in depression. The original treatments were given without anaesthetic. Ostensibly to 'treat' disturbed behaviour, its application, and the threat of it, was undoubtedly sometimes misused as punishment. Sensationalist and misleading portrayals, such as the unmodified ECT given to Jack Nicholson in *One Flew Over the Cuckoo's Nest*, continued to fan the controversy.

In many countries ECT is almost impossible to obtain in public psychiatry – in Italy and Greece and Spain for instance and in California in the US. In England and several US states a ban has been proposed several times but not legislated. Some of this is undoubtedly because of its earlier overuse – many of its fiercest critics are people who received it inappropriately without benefit. However, even for those who support it, there is something very off-putting about it. It seems such a 'crude' assault on that most delicate and important of our organs, the brain. ECT is experienced as an affront to our nature as creative and sentient beings – particularly so as we really do not know how it works. It is vigorously opposed by groups such as the Church of Scientology.

Even more shocking than the overuse of ECT was the crusade of brain surgery conducted by Watts and Freeman in the early 1950s in the US. Brain surgery in psychiatry followed the observation of a freak accident in a Pittsburgh steel mill where a foreman, Phineas Gage, survived a bar passing through his head. The only damage noted was some change in personality – he became more easy-going (but also a bit more disinhibited and foul-mouthed). Severing the connections to the front part of the brain (where the bar had passed) was tried as a last-ditch attempt to reduce intolerable chronic anxiety or disturbed behaviour. It is called leucotomy in Europe and lobotomy in the US and was introduced by a Portuguese psychiatrist Egon Moniz in 1935. He received the Nobel Prize for it in 1949 and, in an ironic twist of fate, was shot dead by a disgruntled patient in 1955.

Psychosurgery probably can help a very limited group of individuals absolutely disabled with severe obsessive compulsive disorder or chronic depression. It appears to work by making the patient uninterested in their symptoms, rather than abolishing them. The patient experiences the obsessional thoughts but doesn't ruminate on them and is able to ignore them. There are changes in personality with the operation – the patient is said to become somewhat 'blunted'.

Brain surgery evokes the same disquiet as ECT. It seems altogether too invasive and brutal. The explanation of how it works is superficial and unconvincing. Freeman and Watts developed a very simple version of the operation that only required a local anaesthetic. Playing down the risks, they travelled across the US carrying out thousands of these operations in large mental hospitals. Between 1939 and 1951 over 50,000 such operations were performed in the US, 3,439 by Freeman alone. Modern techniques are very different (usually involving the destruction of a couple of cubic millimetres of brain tissue) and highly regulated. Only a couple of dozen operations a year are conducted in the UK and the same number in the US. Nevertheless it remains a highly charged issue and one where people rarely change their opinions.

Political abuse in psychiatry

Psychiatry has always had twin obligations – care for the individual patient and protection of society. This 'social control' aspect has to be weighed carefully against individual rights, especially in compulsory treatment. The balance remains a hotly debated issue in most countries. The vastly differing psychiatric care offered to blacks in South Africa under apartheid and in the US Southern States during segregation has often been characterized as political abuse. Similarly the high rate of compulsory detention of ethnic minority patients (particularly blacks of African and Caribbean origin) in England has been cited as an intolerance of different cultures that borders on the repressive. This is probably 'politics with a small p'. Inequitable access to care is a characteristic of many health care systems. It may be inexcusable but it is hardly a deliberate policy aimed at persecuting a specific group.

The use of psychiatry explicitly to repress or silence dissident political opinions in the former Soviet Union was, however, conscious persecution. The Soviets used a diagnosis of 'sluggish schizophrenia'; meaning withdrawal and strangeness which developed slowly without positive symptoms (hallucinations, thought disorder, etc.). Sluggish schizophrenia was used to detain people with dissident political views who opposed the state but demonstrated no clear signs of mental illness. Of course some mentally ill individuals do oppose the state which they believe is persecuting them. The Soviets incarcerated vast numbers of clearly healthy individuals in their forensic psychiatric clinics. This was a scandal that has seriously damaged psychiatry's credibility (particularly in Central and Eastern Europe).

One positive outcome of the Soviet psychiatric abuses was the development of an international movement within psychiatry to challenge such practices. United Nations and Red Cross organizations regularly visit and monitor prisons and detention centres throughout the world and now routinely include mental hospitals in their work. China has recently had to submit to international scrutiny over its dealings with the Falun Gong sect. International awareness provides the strongest protection against political abuse.

Psychiatry unlimited: a diagnosis for everything

Psychiatry has moved centre stage in public health. Four mental illnesses rank in the World Health Organization's top ten global causes of lifelong disability. Depression is currently number two and predicted to be the number one by 2020. Forty-four million Americans have been treated for depression. Is this good news or bad news? It could be a long-overdue recognition of the burden of mental illness as reduced stigma improves detection and recording (and presumably treatment and recovery). Alternatively, it could be that modern living and an ageing population is associated with greater stresses and more mental illnesses. However, rates for established severe mental illnesses such as schizophrenia and bipolar disorder appear static.

Could the rise in mental illness be illusory? Are there other factors at play and could psychiatry go astray if we don't keep an eye on them? Psychiatry operates now in vastly different circumstances from those in which it originated. Medicine enters the 21st century well equipped to detect and control the failings of the early 20th century (professional arrogance and ignorance). Current risks may, however, stem more from psychiatrists unwittingly acting out the agendas of others (as Foucault has insisted they always have). Who else has an agenda?

The patient

Psychiatric diagnoses arise in a dialogue between patient and doctor. The patient offers his concerns and the psychiatrist tests these against the range of illnesses he or she knows. Both parties in this exchange can influence the threshold for what is 'psychiatric'. How do we as individuals interpret our experiences? What do we just accept (even if unpleasant and difficult) and what do we consider unacceptable, worthy of reporting and needing help? We seek help much more readily now and seek it from professionals where previously we might have put up with it or turned to friends and relatives. Anxieties over child-rearing, disappointments in relationships, bereavement, and distress after trauma – all are now considered legitimate territory for psychiatric assessment and possible intervention.

Society has rejected the stiff upper lip and embraced psychology and psychotherapy. It has become immeasurably more tolerant and decent as a result. Our emotions and inner life are taken seriously, we are expected to share them and 'understand our feelings'.

Consequently we seek help with understanding them and relief from them if they become unbearable.

These changes have led to an enormous rise in demand for counselling and psychotherapy and also for antidepressants and medications to reduce anxiety. Of the antidepressants prescribed in the UK 96 per cent are prescribed by family doctors. Most of these are for individuals who will never see a psychiatrist and many who would hardly have been considered unwell a generation earlier. This is not all a bad thing – many patients benefit from these treatments. But there are risks. As treatment thresholds get lower there is less risk that patients who need treatment will be neglected but an increased risk that others who won't benefit do get treatments. Relying on medicines for relief may also inhibit us exploring alternative strategies. Persisting with an unhappy marriage and hoping that the pills will make it better is not a sensible long-term strategy. Similarly our expectations change imperceptibly and personal resilience may be eroded.

Treatments we seek from psychiatrists may even make us worse. Excessive prescription of valium and other sedatives led to an epidemic of dependence which proved enormously difficult to reverse. Some studies indicate that routine counselling after severe road traffic accidents or after stillbirths may *slow down* recovery, not just not help. Perhaps some experiences are best simply put behind one and forgotten. In natural disasters, providing counselling may distract energy and resources from the promotion of self-help and social cohesion.

'Big Pharma'

There is a growing unease about the relationship of the medical profession with the companies which research, manufacture and sell the drugs we use. The cost of developing a prescription drug in the US is estimated at $800,000,000. So the pharmaceutical industry is increasingly concentrated in a small group of immensely powerful multinational businesses. The statistics are staggering. It takes on average up to 10 years from isolating and patenting a molecule, through tests and trials to its first routine prescriptions to patients. Only 1 per cent of new molecules make it from test tube to prescription. The research and development budget is consequently enormous. That of Pfizer (the largest pharmaceutical company in 2005) is greater than the whole national research budget of some European states.

Not surprising then that the marketing of these drugs is ruthless. The financial relationships between doctors and these companies are murky. Over half of all educational meetings for psychiatrists in the US are funded by pharmaceutical companies and luxurious hospitality and travel are routinely offered to doctors as barely concealed inducement for them to prescribe. Until recently psychiatry was immune from this as our drugs cost so little. However the new generation antipsychotics and antidepressants are vastly more expensive (newer 'atypical' antipsychotics cost $2000–$3,000 a year per patient in the US compared to $100–$200 or less for the older drugs; newer antidepressants also cost several hundred dollars a year as opposed to 'pennies' for the old antidepressants such as tofranil and amitryptiline). The patent on a new drug is strictly time limited and the companies have to recoup all their development costs usually within 10–15 years from launch. With the financial muscle of the pharmaceutical companies brought to bear on the profession it is hardly surprising that social and psychological interventions (which have no such financial backing) have a lower profile.

'Big Pharma' has been accused of stretching the boundaries of what are treatable psychiatric disorders to increase the sales of its drugs. It has been accused of creating a need for its drugs rather than developing drugs for existing needs. The enormous success of prozac has lead to an expansion of the concept of clinical depression. Milder and milder cases get treated. Prozac's iconic status has helped reduce stigma against depression but has made it a 'lifestyle' drug. Most university students will know class-mates on antidepressants – inconceivable only a generation ago. Diagnostic patterns have changed in response to the marketing of these drugs. There has been a striking increase in the diagnosis of disorders such as PTSD (post-traumatic stress disorder) and social phobia (a disorder which some would consider just extreme shyness) since drugs have been licensed to treat them.

Even more worrying is the massive growth in psychiatric prescribing for children. Once a rarity, child psychiatrists now regularly prescribe psychotropic drugs for children. The most dramatic increase has been in the diagnosis and treatment of ADHD (attention deficit hyperactivity disorder): 7 per cent of US schoolchildren are diagnosed with ADHD (one in ten boys as they are three times more likely to be diagnosed), with half of these on stimulant drugs.

The prescribing of ritalin (methylphenidate) increased sixfold in the 1990s in the US and accounts for 85 per cent of world prescriptions but Europe is rapidly catching up (150,000 prescriptions in the UK in 2002). Child psychiatrists insist that the diagnosis is made carefully and that drugs are used only after psychological treatments have been tried but the figures simply don't stack up. Irrespective of the controversy about the legitimacy of the diagnosis, there can be little doubt that this is an example of psychiatric practice being rushed by commercial agendas.

Before leaving the pharmaceutical industry we need to acknowledge its very positive contribution to human health and welfare. It would be naïve to ignore the financial imperatives that flow from such staggering R&D costs and to profess surprise at the marketing practices. The dramatic increase in both its scale and power, however, raises ethical problems which are not restricted to psychiatry. They include the exploitation of poorer countries for research where ethical standards may be less strict and where the patients in their trials may never have the resources to benefit from the drugs developed. The temptation to create spurious health needs to sell products is particularly potent in the psychological sphere as almost everyone would like to 'feel a bit better'. Honest debate and tighter guidelines are needed.

Reliability versus validity

Diagnosis in psychiatry has moved towards a criterion-based system (see the diagnostic criteria for depression in Chapter 1). The traditional approach of pattern recognition and reflective empathy informed by extensive familiarity with normal and abnormal behaviours has been replaced by a process of carefully listing features of the disorder that are present. The change was a response to unacceptable variations in diagnostic practice. The new diagnostic system (laid out in the Diagnostic and Statistical Manual – DSM III, now DSM IV) also strove to avoid relying on the psychiatric theories which had caused such conflicts in the past. Whether one really can have an entirely 'atheoretical' diagnostic system is, of course, open to debate.

The new system emphasizes *reliability* (i.e. ensuring that different psychiatrists faced with the same symptoms will always come to the same diagnosis) more than it does *validity* (i.e. ensuring that patients with a particular diagnosis will have similar outcomes and responses to treatment). The goal would be, of course, maximal reliability and maximal validity. Good reliability does not, however, necessarily guarantee good validity. The fact that we all agree on the defining characteristics doesn't mean it really is 'something'. For example, 17th-century witch-finders were very reliable – they all agreed on the tell-tale signs and so consistently agreed on who was a witch before they burnt her. We would not now say that they had really 'identified' a witch, because we don't believe in them, but their methods were certainly very reliable.

Reliability can mistakenly imply validity so that a condition gets accorded the status of a diagnosis essentially because psychiatrists can agree on how to define and recognize it. I have already mentioned a couple of these controversial diagnoses – social phobia and ADHD – but there are several more which really stretch credibility. Nicotine and caffeine 'use disorders' are now both official psychiatric disorders, but few of us would consider these mental illnesses. Similarly there is a range of behavioural patterns which have acquired the highly questionable status of a diagnosis (and therefore may receive 'treatment'). An example is adolescent 'oppositional defiant disorder', which is suspiciously close to the description of a difficult teenager who simply refuses to do what his parents want.

Psychiatric gullibility

Psychiatrists on the whole are trusting souls. They tend to take their patients' stories at face value. This was vividly demonstrated by the psychologist David L. Rosenham's famous study, 'Being Sane in Insane Places'. In 1973 he got eight volunteers to go to emergency rooms in America complaining of a voice in their head which said 'empty', 'hollow', or 'thud'. All eight were admitted to psychiatric units where they then behaved absolutely normally. The most amazing thing was that they stayed in hospital for an average of just under three weeks each before they were discharged. Even worse, most of them got a diagnosis on discharge of 'schizophrenia in remission'. Not surprising then that there is such a call for reliability.

So there are several forces acting on psychiatry (including the natural curiosity of researchers) which threaten continued expansion. Whether this is a desirable development is one that should not be left to the profession alone to decide but requires debate within the broader society (i.e. you).

Personality problems and addictions

Psychiatrists have always dealt with the consequences of drug and alcohol addictions. They have also always recognized that there are groups of individuals whose personalities are markedly abnormal and can cause endless problems. The degree of human misery associated with these problems is beyond dispute, and such

DSM IV Diagnostic criteria for Oppositional Defiant Disorder

A. A pattern of negativistic, hostile, and defiant behaviour lasting at least 6 months, during which four (or more) of the following are present:

often loses temper

often argues with adults

often actively defies or refuses to comply with adults' requests or rules

often deliberately annoys people

often blames others for his or her mistakes or misbehaviour

is often touchy or easily annoyed by others

is often angry and resentful

is often spiteful or vindictive

Note: consider a criterion met only if the behaviour occurs more frequently than is typically observed in individuals of comparable age and developmental level.

B. The disturbance in behaviour causes clinically significant impairment in social, academic, or occupational functioning.

C. The behaviours do not occur exclusively during the course of a Psychotic or Mood Disorder.

D. Criteria are not met for Conduct Disorder, and, if the individual is age 18 years or older, criteria are not met for Antisocial Personality Disorder.

individuals are found in large numbers in mental health services. There are, however, strong arguments for and against whether these are *primarily* psychiatric disorders and whether psychiatrists should be responsible for treating them. This is no simple academic argument that could allow both sides to just make individual decisions that suit them. People with these problems may be, and are, treated against their wishes.

Coercion in psychiatry

Compulsory treatment is permitted in psychiatry in every society – including Western societies whose very founding principles are respect for individual liberty before the law. This very striking exception stems from the observation that during periods of illness an individual's judgement is impaired and they are not able to make rational decisions; mental illnesses often involve a 'break' with normal functioning and a change that estranges the patient from their normal self. Unlike, for instance, a learning disability where the individual may also not be able to make informed and rational decisions because they have never developed the capacity, the striking characteristic of mental illnesses is the *change*. Most societies have sanctioned a paternalistic provision for coercive treatment from a humane desire to protect an individual who is clearly 'not themselves'. This resolve is strengthened by the repeated observation that patients recover and express the same concerns as the rest of us about their behaviour when unwell. Many are even grateful that they were forcibly treated.

Lawyers find these areas difficult. The standard assessment of 'capacity' to make treatment decisions (the ability to *understand* the information, the ability to *trust* the individual giving the information, and the ability to *retain* and make a decision based on that information) works well for children, the learning disabled, and those with dementia. However, it doesn't work well where the problem is one of judgement and mood rather than intellectual ability. Imposing treatment against a patient's will rests ultimately on the psychiatrist's conclusion that the patient is suffering from a mental illness such that their current decisions are not those they would usually express. Note that this involves the psychiatrist making a judgement on what he believes that the patient would *usually do* or want when well. Compulsion is also sometimes used as a brief safety measure with people who are 'temporarily unbalanced' – a terrified individual in a strange place or young people attempting to kill or harm themselves in despair after a relationship break-up.

Severe personality disorders

Psychiatry's attitude to psychopathic and antisocial personality disorder usually in men, and borderline personality disorder, usually in women, presents ethical and conceptual concerns. Psychopaths are cold, callous individuals who lack empathy for others and consequently can commit awful crimes. They give no thought to the consequences for others and show no remorse afterwards. They are often recognizable early on (death of pets, arson, etc.). Being self-centred and not caring about others' feelings they can be extremely successful; it is jokingly proposed that mild psychopathy is an essential for being a successful politician. Psychopaths are often lumped together with explosive and violent individuals as antisocial personality disorder. This group is a massive problem for the prisons and criminal justice system.

In some countries psychiatrists detain these individuals under the same conditions as the mentally ill and this has been criticized as an abuse of power. Compulsory treatment is justified mainly by the belief that the patient is not making the decisions that they would normally make and which they will make again after recovery. To warrant coercion the condition is usually time-limited and it is believed with some confidence that the treatment will speed recovery. None of these conditions are met for severe personality disorders. Their behaviour reflects their personality – their real identity; they are not aberrant or temporary, and to date there is no convincing evidence that forced treatments will significantly change them.

Such people pose profound challenges for society. They have often committed serious sexual and violent crimes and it is obvious to prison staff that, as little has changed, they will offend again. In England they are labelled as having a dangerous severe personality disorder (DSPD) and highly staffed new units have been built to treat them. But is their potentially indefinite detention by psychiatrists (as opposed to a prison sentence when they break the law) any less an abuse than the detention of political prisoners in the Soviet system was? The humanitarian sentiments of those involved do not remove the ethical dilemma.

The Western world has experienced an upsurge in chaotic self-damaging behaviour in young women. Overdosing and cutting have become common features of female inmates of mental hospitals and prisons. Patients seem out of control, are clearly distressed, and damage themselves in what often seems like a mixture of anger and a desperate plea for help. Psychiatrists feel responsible but impotent and often try to 'contain' the situation by keeping the patient compulsorily on a ward offering supervision and support. Unfortunately things may go from bad to worse – the patient self-harms more and the psychiatrist increases the restrictions to control the situation. A vociferous pressure group argues that what these women do to their bodies is their own affair and psychiatry is overstepping the mark in treating them against their will. They point to the cultural precedents for self-mutilation (religious and ritual scarring are common in many societies) and underline how medicine, and psychiatry in particular, has consistently denied women's self-determination over their own bodies.

Drug and alcohol abuse

A similar set of arguments holds for drug and alcohol abuse. Both can be associated with mental illness and both can also cause mental illnesses. Fine for psychiatry to be involved then. But are drug or alcohol abuse mental illnesses in themselves? The rebranding of addictions as illnesses was a humanitarian impulse in the 1940s after the founding of Alcoholics Anonymous in 1939, to provide help to detoxify addicted individuals and support sobriety. The world's largest self-help groups (Alcoholics Anonymous, AA, and Narcotics Anonymous, NA) both consider addiction a lifelong illness, although they rely on personal and spiritual support rather than medical treatment.

AA and NA view the addict as fundamentally different from other individuals, never able to use drugs or alcohol sensibly. Within psychiatry, however, there are divided views. Many view addiction as an illness to be treated like any other mental disorder. Others see drug and alcohol abuse as dangerous habits that can lead to mental illnesses but are not themselves illnesses, and ultimately are the responsibility of the individuals themselves. The medicalization of substance abuse is criticized as a distraction from effective public health measures such as raising the price and restricting access. Both of the latter have been shown to reduce drinking and drink-related illnesses and deaths.

Offering help such as prescribing medicines to cope with withdrawal and support to build up a sober lifestyle are uncontroversial. Concerns arise from the use of compulsion which is common to a limited degree in most countries. In much of Scandinavia, Eastern Europe, and Russia, however, there has been extensive use of specialized mental hospitals for longer term detention and treatment of alcoholics and drug addicts. Can this be justified? The consequences of heavy drinking or drug abuse can undoubtedly be disastrous, even fatal. But many of us make foolish decisions and suffer the consequences – smoking is probably more dangerous than drinking but we don't compulsorily treat smokers. The confused thinking and poor judgement when intoxicated is also a questionable justification for psychiatric intervention as the express purpose of becoming intoxicated is to alter judgements by blurring an unattractive reality.

Increasing sophistication in genetics and epidemiology has helped identify those who are at greater risk of alcoholism and drug abuse.

There are well recognized ethnic variations in the ability to tolerate and metabolize alcohol. These findings strengthen the contention that these are not simply personal choices but disorders, much in the same way that schizophrenia is a disorder – we just don't yet know as much about it as we do about schizophrenia. Some even propose that self-destructive drinking and drug use *must* be the result of a mental illness. Clearly the issue is still open and psychiatric engagement with drug and alcohol abusing patients will continue to attract some controversy.

The insanity defence

The coercion controversies in psychiatry are about unfairly depriving individuals of their rights. An important motive in early mental health legislation, however, was to protect patients from being punished for crimes they committed when unwell. Society has always felt uncomfortable about such punishments. The crime of infanticide was distinguished from murder because 19th-century juries refused to convict and send to the hangman mothers who killed their babies while suffering post-partum psychoses.

The importance of establishing criminal intent ('mens rea' or 'guilty mind') has guaranteed a long and tortured relationship between psychiatrists and the courts. Agreeing whether or not someone was insane at the time of the crime (i.e. unable to judge the significance of their acts and realize that they were wrong) has in principle been fairly straightforward. However it is often far from easy in the individual case. Similarly floridly ill patients, unable fully to understand what is going on in court, may be judged unfit to plead and admitted to hospital for treatment. Most countries will accept the decision of unfit to plead on the basis of a psychiatric assessment or will return a not-guilty verdict on the grounds of insanity.

The real problems in court concern diminished responsibility on the grounds of mental illness – particularly where the criminal behaviour itself is the clearest manifestation of the disorder. It is less a problem with a grossly disturbed individual whose crime is just one among many signs of the illness (such as a manic patient in court for reckless driving but who also at that time is not sleeping, dressing in outrageous clothes, and spending all his money). Proposing personality disorders as a defence (i.e. because a psychopath does not notice or care about the distress caused) strikes at the concept of free will and personal responsibility that is the very foundation of criminal justice systems. Most criminals have had dreadful childhoods. Many have been abused. Few have skilled jobs or stable families to fall back upon. So it is not surprising that we may temper justice with mercy. But is there not a circularity in citing the very qualities that give rise to the crime as an excuse for a reduced punishment? This ethical dilemma is particularly sharp in individuals with Asperger's syndrome (a mild form of autism) who cannot see the world from the other's perspective and cannot interpret others' motives even though they may desperately want to.

In practice the more serious the crime and the greater the risk, the easier the decision. Where the alternative to a guilty verdict and prison is hospital care (and sometimes secure hospital care) courts and juries feel more comfortable to make the allowance. In lesser cases, where punishment is not so severe, and might just deter a repetition, it is argued that a psychiatric defence is unjustified and probably does the individual no favours in the long term. Thomas Szasz (Chapter 5) insists that the psychiatric defence is a denial of the fundamental rights and obligations of the individual. A psychiatric defence is generally accepted for individuals where the disorder is plainly there for all to see.

Sometimes the only evidence of a disorder is the crime. There have been several high-profile cases of murder where the perpetrator denies any memory, claiming it occurred during an 'automatism' (a dream-like or dissociated state). In even more extreme cases 'multiple personalities' have been proposed where a single individual has several fully developed identities, each completely independent of each other. This is a very attractive concept which captures the popular imagination (e.g. Robert Louis Stevenson's 1885 novel *Dr Jekyll and Mr Hyde*, and the 1957 film *The Three Faces of Eve*).

The postulated mechanism is that some mental functioning is so successfully repressed that it is only accessible through deep psychotherapy or 'triggered' in highly specific situations. This is of enormous psychiatric/legal significance in cases of alleged childhood sexual abuse. The extent to which children are exposed to sexual abuse by family members has long been controversial in psychiatry. The pendulum has swung back and forth between considering it a common trauma that causes neuroses to the alternative belief that it is rare and most reports are 'false memories' arising from current distress and confusion. Currently the presumption is in favour of believing the adult who complains of child sexual abuse. This has resulted in high-profile cases splitting families when 'recovered memories' have been unearthed. Psychiatrists appear on both sides of the case, stressing either the damaging impact of abuse, repressed over many years, or, conversely, the patient's suggestibility in over-enthusiastic therapy.

Psychiatry: a controversial practice

Psychiatric practice will probably always be risky and controversial. Many psychiatrists argue for a more limited approach, restricting it to clearly identifiable and agreed mental illnesses: 'We should stick to treating diagnosed illnesses, schizophrenia, anorexia nervosa, depression and accept that there are many other causes of human distress beyond mental illness.' 'We should leave the social policy and ethics to the politicians and philosophers.' This is an attractive argument. The history of psychiatry is full of examples of over-stepping the mark. But as we have seen in this chapter it is not simply up to the psychiatrists – there are other stakeholders and powerful forces at play with broad ethical issues and significant potential benefits in the balance.

Scientific developments are expanding what we can do; families and patients have steadily rising expectations from us; governments and the pharmaceutical industry challenge us with new demands, inducements, and opportunities. We could only possibly avoid controversy and the risk of potential mistakes if we turned our back on progress and innovation. But that means not fulfilling either psychiatry's promise or its obligations. Straddling hard science and the field of human behaviour and ambitions, it is simply impossible for psychiatry to be uncontroversial. It comes with the territory and, as we are about to explore in Chapter 7, may be getting worse.

Chapter 7
Into the 21st century

New technologies and old dilemmas

> It doesn't matter what he does, he'll never amount to anything.
> (Albert Einstein's teacher, 1895)

> Computers in future may weigh no more than 1.5 tons.
> (Popular Mechanics, 1949)

> We don't like their sound, and guitar music is on the way out.
> (Decca Records on the Beatles, 1962)

It is risky to make predictions. Psychiatry at the beginning of the 21st century is very different to that of just a few decades ago. Who could have imagined that we would be able to visualize not only the living brain's structure in minute detail but even watch as different regions light up with specific emotions or during hallucinations? Could we have foreseen diagnoses derived by computers or psychotherapies on the web with neither psychiatrist nor psychologist involved? Psychiatry is changing and the rate of change intensifies the dilemmas raised in Chapter 6. Optimists believe these will fade away as the scientific base of psychiatry becomes firmer, but there is little evidence for this yet. The areas of concern may shift but they seem, if anything, as pressing.

Improvements in brain science

We will continue to experience an acceleration in our understanding of brain functioning. Neurosciences have become *the* 'hot topic' in biomedical research, driven by increasingly powerful tools for visualizing and measuring brain functioning. For so long it has been a mysterious, apparently inert organ with no moving parts. Modern imaging techniques reveal the brain's dynamism, allowing us to observe activity spread through it with individual areas activating sequentially in response to stimulation. And not just responding to external stimuli, but solving mathematical problems or even discriminating between pictures of people we like or don't like.

The big leap forward came with imaging. The structure of the brain has been studied in great detail by anatomists for over a century. They identified the function of areas by examining the brains of people who had had strokes and lost different functions. Shrinkage or damage to the brain could be demonstrated in post-mortems and by x-ray techniques. These later involved either injecting dye into the bloodstream or air into the ventricles (fluid-filled cavities that exist normally in the brain). Visualization of the body's structures took a great leap forward with CAT scanning and then MRI scanning. These use magnetic fields to produce amazingly detailed images of 'slices' through any part of the body (including the brain) that can be used to construct 3D pictures. While these techniques were useful in diagnosing brain tumours and demonstrating dementia they were of little help in most psychiatric disorders. Indeed, the term 'functional disorder' has long been used as shorthand for psychiatric illnesses precisely because no structural abnormalities could be shown.

Functional imaging has been a further advance for psychiatry. There are already three different types – measuring increased blood flow, measuring cell metabolism with the use of marked chemicals,

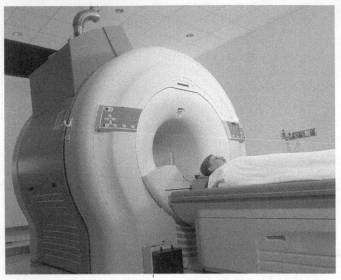

14. MRI scanner: the first really detailed visualization of the brain's structure

and now even directly measuring the electric activity of nerve cells. We can now show that thinking and feeling are reflected in activities in different parts of the brain and that the same parts of the brain are active when patients hallucinate as when we hear real voices. Functional imaging has confirmed the complexity and interconnectedness of brain activity.

Have these imaging techniques changed psychiatry yet? They have certainly increased knowledge and helped us understand the biochemical systems in the brain associated with disorders, and this has improved drug research. There are, as yet, no major advances in clinical practice as a direct result. Some early experiments are under way to transplant brain cells in Parkinson's disease into areas where activity has been demonstrated to be deficient. There has even been a trial of inserting minuscule 'batteries' into the brains of some people with chronic depression to

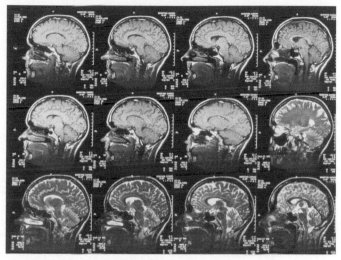

15. A series of brain pictures from a single MRI scan. Each picture is a 'slice' through the brain structure, from which a 3D image can be constructed

sec if they stimulate an increased release of transmitter substances and alleviate the depression.

This is a long way from the 'Cyborg' fantasy of so many films where small computer chips are inserted into the brain and control behaviour. There is a noticeable reluctance among neuroscientists to develop brain interventions for mental illnesses. Interfering directly with an individual's consciousness and taking it out of their control generates strong resistance in scientists, as in the rest of us. This is in contrast, however, to surgery and cell transplantation in brain diseases such as Parkinson's disease, which do not have the same implications for selfhood.

The human genome and genetic research

Ever since Crick and Watson clarified the double helix structure of DNA in 1953 genetic research has been in overdrive. Genetics used to be the territory of plant and animal breeders applying Mendel's laws, and medical researchers tracking familial diseases such as haemophilia and Huntington's disease. Now it has blossomed into a programme which has mapped the very chromosomes and genes themselves. Previously geneticists could only inform patients about their statistical chances of passing on disorders. Now they can know for certain in some cases if the patient is carrying a disorder and even (as in the case of Huntington's disease, a rare distressing disorder with both psychiatric and movement manifestations) predict if an at-risk individual will develop it years in the future.

Not many psychiatric disorders, however, have simple 'Mendelian' genetic patterns where half (dominant) or a quarter (recessive) of the offspring are destined to have the illness. Most of the major disorders (e.g. schizophrenia, bipolar disorder) do run in families and have an undeniable genetic component but there are almost certainly several genes involved and they have been very difficult to identify. There have been many false dawns. Currently the likeliest candidate is Neuregulin 1 (a gene identified in schizophrenia families in Iceland and the West of Scotland). However this gene is more widespread than is schizophrenia – possibly up to 30 per cent of the population may carry it. Neuregulin 1 appears to be *necessary* for developing schizophrenia, but not *sufficient*. Some life experiences (or perhaps combination with other genes) are also required. So an interaction between nature and nurture is indicated. This may explain why the issue has been so resistant to the 'either—or' solutions of the past. It holds out hope that even in those with the genes for the disorder it may be possible to prevent schizophrenia developing.

While genetic research has yet to have a major clinical impact, in practice it has certainly stirred up thinking. What level of risk are we willing to take if we know that we have a higher than average chance of our child developing schizophrenia or depression? Would it be ethically acceptable to start screening for these disorders once the genes have been confidently identified? What if we were also able to identify genes for being clever – would it be OK to screen for that? Screening implies selection. It is usually only done if the individual wants to know whether to start or continue with a pregnancy.

Early identification

These problems already confront some families with schizophrenia. An Australian service for treating young people with schizophrenia as early as possible has begun successfully to identify individuals who are at very high risk of developing the illness. These are usually adolescents in families with schizophrenic members and who themselves are 'odd' or 'withdrawn' and report unusual, but not clearly psychotic, experiences. Should the team, being fairly certain that the young person is likely to become ill, offer treatment with antipsychotic drugs? They have conducted a trial where they gave one half drugs and the other half placebo. Those given drugs developed fewer psychoses. However, not all of those without drugs did become ill (i.e. if it had not been a trial they could have been given the drugs unnecessarily). The implications for young people at such a sensitive stage of their development are clearly enormous. This is just one example of the sort of decisions we will increasingly face as technologies improve.

Specificity of gene identification in mental illness is still a long way off. Any large-scale genetic screening to avoid psychiatric disorders would inevitably mean a steady reduction in the rich variety of human behaviour. How happy would we be with that – a world without Van Gogh or without Schumann?

Brainwashing and thought control

Most of the scarier fantasies about psychiatry have usually been about its 'awesome powers'. Ever since the term 'brainwashing' was first used during the Korean War in the 1950s these fears have condensed around it. In truth psychiatrists have little extra knowledge about such procedures beyond those well known in cognitive and group psychology. Psychiatrists and psychologists do advise governments and the military about how to persuade people but their techniques are hardly more advanced (if *as* advanced) as those of successful advertising agencies.

Millgram's famous experiment is mistakenly quoted as an example of this power. He used actors to demonstrate that normal people were prepared to deliver severe, even life-threatening, electrical shocks to other people if told it was part of a psychology experiment. This study did not demonstrate the awesome power of psychology, but rather the scarier, but commonplace, propensity we all have to surrender our judgement to 'authorities'.

Where some of the earlier 'science fiction' fantasies have proved right is in the pervasive use of mood-altering drugs. 'Soma' in Aldous Huxley's novel *Brave New World* was a drug to keep the masses contented and submissive in a totalitarian state. How far are we from that when 30 per cent of the adult population of France were taking psychiatric drugs in the late 1990s and when 10 per cent (and rising) of US schoolboys are taking ritalin? There is an increasing availability of such drugs which both treat mental illness and also enhance how healthy people feel. 'Better than well' is how many describe the effects of these 'designer' drugs. People have always self-medicated with recreational drugs but now prescribed drugs are widely used to deal with normal life stresses.

This risk that psychiatry may invade all aspects of our life and 'medicalize' the human condition is increased by the emphasis on the simpler, more reliable but democratically negotiated approach to diagnosis discussed in Chapter 6. The size of the psychiatric population used to be restricted by psychiatrists only giving a diagnosis when the patient's experience and behaviour was felt to be fundamentally 'different'. If a diagnosis follows automatically from a series of complaints (without being filtered through such a judgement) then there is little restriction on expansion. We increasingly encourage self-disclosure and attention to our feelings, hence perhaps the rapidly rising number of people who consider themselves depressed or anxious. Most of us welcome this more accepting, open approach to human experience. Equally, most of us support a more balanced relationship embodied in a psychiatric consultation which takes the patient's symptoms more seriously than the psychiatrist's preoccupations. But are we happy with the consequences as ever-increasing segments of our lives become labelled as psychiatric disorder?

Old dilemmas in new forms

Despite all this we enter the 21st century with remarkably similar dilemmas with which we entered the 20th. Compulsion in psychiatry has not gone away – rather increased somewhat. Similarly the fear that psychiatry may trivialize individual differences and treat people as objects remains just as strong. This conflict may now be played out between 'evidence based medicine' versus 'post-modern individualism', where once it was the crushing uniformity of large asylums versus the dignity of the patient. Society and psychiatry will always have (and probably *should* always have) an uneasy relationship balancing duty to the patients and duty to society in the social control of a small number of potentially dangerous individuals. The very durability of these debates reveals them as not simply technical problems. They reflect the tensions and paradoxes that are inherent to psychiatry as a discipline and with which we started this book.

Will psychiatry survive the 21st century?

The imminent demise of psychiatry has been predicted for most of its history. Optimists (particularly those engaged in medical and biological research) anticipate dramatic breakthroughs that will tame mental illnesses in the way that antibiotics defeated tuberculosis or vaccination eradicated small pox. The mental hygiene movement also hoped that rational child care, reduced alcohol consumption, and improved social conditions would make the analyst and psychotherapist redundant. It hasn't happened so far. The very success of modern medicine has brought with it the challenges of an ageing population with increased depression and Alzheimer's disease. Greater openness and respect for individual feelings has resulted in an enormous increase in the demand for counselling and psychotherapy. The numbers of psychiatrists and mental health professionals has risen inexorably across the world. On a simple head-count of staff and the mounting demand for its service, yes it should continue to flourish.

But will it survive as it is now? Certainly things are changing. Might the psychological and psychotherapeutic treatments separate from the more traditionally medical treatment of the psychoses? In many parts of the world psychiatry has only recently gained its independence from neurology but we now hear strong calls for reuniting them as a logical development of a more powerful medical psychiatry for the future. Many psychiatrists already call themselves 'neuropsychiatrists'. This is the case in many Germanic systems. There are several health care systems where the psychiatrists deal with diagnosis and inpatient care, emphasizing a highly scientific medical model. Long-term outpatient care of disabled patients is managed by social workers and psychologists/psychotherapists using a more interpersonal approach. These pressures are not new. What is new is the wide availability of highly trained clinical psychologists, nurses, and social workers with the necessary skills. Responsibilities and power structures are shifting and radically different practices evolving.

There is a logic to such developments. Increased knowledge drives specialization, so some fragmentation of psychiatry is inevitable. Despite this, psychiatry is entrenching as a discipline. Establishing departments of psychiatry independent of neurology or internal medicine is still seen as a marker of progress. Similarly when people can choose they still seem to want that mixture of medical expertise (or is it authority?) combined with psychological and emotional sensitivity traditional to psychiatry. Psychiatry's medical pedigree gives reassurance yet few of us believe that it is really *just* a branch of medicine.

The mind is not the same as the brain. The defining characteristic of mental illnesses (and consequently psychiatry) remains their impact on our sense of self and on our closest relationships. Working with these is the hallmark of psychiatry and there is no evidence of society losing interest in it. There probably will be a *Very Short Introduction to Psychiatry* in a hundred years' time.

Further reading

This VSI has been a whirlwind tour round psychiatry. It *does not* aim to give a technical or professional understanding of the subject, nor to give advice about what to do for a psychiatric problem you think you or someone close to you may have. Hopefully you will feel able to approach a professional and will realize that there is a tolerant and welcoming reception for you if you do. Here are a few suggestions for those who want to read more.

Chapter 1

Gelder, M., Mayou, R., and Geddes, J., *Psychiatry*, Oxford Core Texts (OUP, 2005)

There are several textbooks of psychiatry but even the best of them is written to accompany practical training and my inclination would not be to recommend one. However if you really do want to look up a specific illness or problem then I would currently recommend a textbook rather than the web, which can be very confusing.

Chapters 2 and 3

Porter, Roy, *Madness: A Brief History* (OUP, 2002)
Shorter, Edward, *A History of Psychiatry* (Wiley, 1997)
Jones, Kathleen, *Asylums and After* (Athlone Press, 1993)

Almost anything by the late Roy Porter is worth reading on the history of asylums (which he called 'museums of madness'). Shorter is even more critical of the profession. Kathleen Jones's book is the classic and most balanced but no longer in print, though obtainable through libraries. All are entertaining but each has a definite perspective.

Chapter 4

Storr, Anthony, *Freud: A Very Short Introduction* (OUP, 2001)
Stevens, Anthony, *Jung: A Very Short Introduction* (OUP, 2001)

These are two short, jargon-free introductions to the two most dominant figures in the psychoanalytical movement.

Chapter 5

Laing, R. D., *The Divided Self* (Penguin Books, 1960)
Foucault, Michel, *Madness and Civilization* (Tavistock Publications, 1961)
Bentall, Richard, *Madness Explained: Psychosis and Human Nature* (Penguin Books, 2003)

The Divided Self is the iconic anti-psychiatry text of the 1960s. Foucault is much harder to read. Bentall brings the debate up to the minute with a more scientific, less philosophical, approach but which is still very challenging. All these books are still in print.

Chapter 6

Porter's and Shorter's books have lots to say about these issues too. Erving Goffman, *Asylums* (1961), is rather long but led the charge against the asylums by exposing malpractice.

Index

Psychiatry

Psychiatry

Index